T0323906

MEDICAL DOCUMENTATION, BILLING, AND CODING FOR THE ADVANCED PRACTICE NURSE

Written specifically for student and new nurse practitioners, this guide presents the essentials of how to document, code, bill, and get reimbursed for services provided in practice.

Coding is a core skill that requires practice and a nurse practitioner is responsible for the accuracy of codes submitted on a claim form. This book covers the context and background for billing and coding, how to document correctly, the 2021/2023 evaluation and management coding changes, specialty services, the legal implications of coding, and medical necessity. Using a *read it, see it, do it* approach as a learning strategy, the book includes case studies from a range of inpatient and outpatient settings and practice exercises to try out your skills. Resources linked to updates on billing and coding rules are provided as an appendix to ensure the content can be applicable long term.

This text is an invaluable resource for students and nurse practitioners new to coding and billing.

Carol Berger is an inspiring, dedicated health professional and teacher. Her credentials include Doctor of Nursing Practice (DNP), Master of Science in Nursing (MSN), and Certified Family Nurse Practitioner. She has devoted her life to serving her patients and students. Currently serving as an Associate Professor of Nursing at the Catherine McAuley School of Nursing within Maryville University's esteemed Myrtle E. and Earl E. Walker College of Health Professions, Dr. Berger brings her life experience as a nurse and provider to inspire and educate the rising generation. She is a co-creator of the website http://simplyaprn.com which contains different lectures on pathophysiology and pharmacology as well as interactive games to reinforce learning concepts for the rising generation of nursing students, as well as co-host of the NP Changing Practice podcast.

Theresa Galakatos is a dynamic and accomplished healthcare professional who has established herself as a prominent figure in the nursing and academic spheres. With an impressive array of credentials, including a Doctor of Nursing Practice (DNP), a Doctor of Philosophy in Nursing (Ph.D.), a Master of Social Work (MSW), and multiple Master of Science in Nursing (MSN) degrees, she stands as a true exemplar of lifelong learning and dedication to the field. Currently serving as an Associate Professor of Nursing at the Catherine McAuley School of Nursing within Maryville University's esteemed Myrtle E. and Earl E. Walker College of Health Professions, Dr. Galakatos brings her wealth of knowledge and practical experience to inspire and educate the next generation of healthcare professionals.

Nina A. Zimmermann is an influential nursing professor and experienced adult gerontology primary care nurse practitioner. She earned her Master of Science in Nursing (MSN) in Nursing Education, a Post-Masters Certificate in Adult-Gerontology Primary Care Nurse Practitioner, and her Doctorate in Education (EdD). She is considered an expert in nursing education and primary care practice. Her current academic position is as Associate Professor of Nursing at the Catherine McAuley School of Nursing within Maryville University's esteemed Myrtle E. and Earl E. Walker College of Health Professions. Dr. Zimmerman contributes her advanced nursing practice experience and nursing education of nurse practitioners to this textbook and to future primary care nurse practitioners.

MEDICAL DOCUMENTATION, BILLING, AND CODING FOR THE ADVANCED PRACTICE NURSE

Carol Berger, Theresa Galakatos, and Nina A. Zimmermann

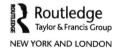

NEW YORK AND LONDON

Cover image: Getty Images

First published 2025
by Routledge
605 Third Avenue, New York, NY 10158

and by Routledge
4 Park Square, Milton Park, Abingdon, Oxon, OX14 4RN

Routledge is an imprint of the Taylor & Francis Group, an informa business

Library of Congress Cataloging-in-Publication Data
Names: Berger, Carol (Carol Ann), author. | Galakatos, Theresa, author. | Zimmerman, Nina A., author.
Title: Medical documentation, billing and coding for the advanced practice nurse / Carol Berger, Theresa Galakatos, and Nina A. Zimmerman.
Description: Abingdon, Oxon ; New York, NY : Routledge, 2025. | Includes bibliographical references and index.
Subjects: MESH: Clinical Coding—methods | Nurse Practitioners | Medical Records | Advanced Practice Nursing | Medical Assistance | United States
Classification: LCC RB115 (print) | LCC RB115 (ebook) | NLM W 80 | DDC 616.0012—dc23/eng/20240813
LC record available at https://lccn.loc.gov/2024033844
LC ebook record available at https://lccn.loc.gov/2024033845

ISBN: 978-1-032-89440-9 (hbk)
ISBN: 978-1-032-89439-3 (pbk)
ISBN: 978-1-003-54287-2 (ebk)

DOI: 10.4324/9781003542872

Typeset in Bembo
by codeMantra

CONTENTS

ABOUT THE AUTHORS

Dr. Carol Berger has 45 years of experience as a nurse working in acute, long-term care, consultant, and case management. As a consultant she found out how important documentation was for reimbursement. Educating nursing staff on documentation was a key part of her consulting role. In 2007, she graduated from the University of Missouri–St. Louis (UMSL) as a Family Nurse Practitioner. As a provider she has worked as a hospitalist and in a rural clinic for 7 years before going into teaching full time. As an educator she serves to inspire and empower her students with a holistic understanding of healthcare.

She obtained her doctorate in 2012 while working in rural health. Dr. Berger became aware of the oral health issues in the community and lack of dental providers in her area. Research from her doctoral project was published in the *Nurse Practitioner* in 2014 – *Oral Health for Children*. Since joining Maryville, she has gone further with her research involving analysis of the entire data set between the years 2013–2016 from the Missouri Oral Health Program showing that the Missouri Oral Health Program was effective. Her research was again published in the *Nurse Practitioner* in 2020 – *Implementation Science: Changing Practice in Oral Health*. A documentary was created in collaboration with Dr. Scott Angus and Lilli Kayes both colleagues earning her the Missouri Oral Health Champion Award in 2022. Dr. Berger is considered an expert in the field of oral health for children, presenting her findings at many conferences and organizations.

She is the lead teacher of Health Promotion for Maryville's graduate program and has incorporated all aspects of holistic health into the program including completing the Life Smiles course which is a national health promotion objective. She has also taught advanced pathophysiology, pharmacology, and leadership. Beyond the classroom, Dr. Berger serves her community. She is truly a role model for all those who know her with the goal of expanding her circle of influence through compassion and healing.

Other publications include *Health Promotions for the Provider* by Kindall and Hunt (2023).

Dr. Theresa Galakatos has an extensive track record of clinical expertise, having served in leadership and clinical positions at renowned medical institutions such as Barnes − Jewish Hospital and Forest Park Hospital. Her commitment to patient care, paired with her passion for teaching, has led her to excel in her academic career. As an Associate Professor, she has been instrumental in shaping the education of nursing students, imparting both practical skills and theoretical knowledge. Her innovative teaching methods, which include incorporating an active learning environment and embracing diverse/inclusive perspectives, have captivated learners and created engaging educational experiences.

Beyond her roles in the classroom, Dr. Galakatos serves as a leader in the local community raising awareness and funding for resources for seniors. She is deeply involved in the academic community. Dr. Galakatos has taken on leadership roles in departmental and university-wide committees, including serving as Chair of the Promotion and Tenure Committee and participating in various curriculum development initiatives. Her dedication extends to mentoring and guiding fellow faculty members, as well as chairing doctoral projects for Doctor of Nursing Practice candidates.

Dr. Galakatos' contributions to research and scholarship are equally impressive. She has published in peer-reviewed journals, presented at conferences, and engaged in community collaborations, showcasing her commitment to advancing nursing practice and patient care. Her remarkable accomplishments have not gone unnoticed, as demonstrated by her recognition with awards such as the Walker Award and the Anna Ikeda-Tabor Nursing Research Award.

In all facets of her career, Dr. Theresa Galakatos exemplifies a tireless pursuit of excellence, a commitment to patient-centered care, and a passion for fostering the growth of future healthcare professionals. Her multifaceted expertise, teaching prowess, and unwavering dedication make her a true luminary in the field of nursing and academia.

Dr. Nina A. Zimmermann is an Assistant Professor of Nursing at Maryville University and an adult nurse practitioner (NP). In 2019, she earned her doctorate in education at Maryville University. Dr. Zimmermann has 15 years of advanced practice nursing and 13 years of nurse practitioner education experience and she is a board-certified adult primary care NP with a primary care clinical practice in St. Louis and Maryville Health and Wellness Clinic. She has published and presented in her research areas of adherence to clinical practice guidelines for asthma, asthma patient and family education, innovative and active-learning online teaching strategies, NP students learning how to document a patient encounter, and the use of infographics to promote nursing students' learning of their patient's culture and diversity. She is a co-host of the Nurse Practitioners Changing Practice podcast and co-creator of the website https://simplyaprn.com/

PREFACE

This book is for nurse practitioner (NP) students and all health-care providers who seek a comprehensive guide regarding billing and coding. We dedicate this book to our current and previous NP students as well as our students who have become trustworthy and dedicated healthcare providers. We acknowledge and appreciate our Psychiatric Mental Health NP colleague, Dr. Brandie Smalley, and her contribution to the psychiatric and mental health documentation included in this book. This book is a product of Dr. Carol Berger's mission and vision as an NP educator and healthcare provider. The co-authors greatly appreciate Dr. Carol Berger's knowledge and expertise, attention to detail, persistence, friendship, and guidance for us to collectively write, edit and complete this book.

Dr. Carol Berger
Dr. Theresa Galakatos
Dr. Nina A. Zimmermann

THE HISTORY OF MEDICARE
AND MEDICAID

In 1965, President Lyndon B. Johnson signed into law the Social Security Amendment which gave birth to Medicare and Medicaid. However, efforts for a national healthcare system for United States (US) citizens started early in the twentieth century. Government concern over sickness and lost wages began in 1911. *Sickness insurance* was the insurance proposed at the time with the goal of reimbursement for some of the lost wages and medical expenses of workers who became ill. This bill was modeled after the British National Insurance Act of 1911. The British National Insurance Act secured a cash benefit to workers for up to 26 weeks (about 6 months). The only problem with this insurance was it only covered workers and not their families or people who were not employed. Rubinow (1916), a healthcare reformer, noted that US wages lost by the labor force exceeded medical costs, citing a study completed in 1911. He concentrated on getting sickness insurance laws through the states due to the constraints on federal activity and because of the belief that states would know better than the federal government what their populations needed. The sickness insurance plan was debated in places that were heavily populated such as New York and California but despite such debate the measure was defeated in every state that brought it for a vote (Hirshfield, 1970). The American Medical Association (AMA) did not back this bill, citing that "*medical care was a private transaction between a medical practitioner and a patient*"

DOI: 10.4324/9781003542872-1

(Berkowitz, 2005–2006). Medical doctors had a fear of being legislated in their treatment decisions and did not want national health insurance interfering with their ability to practice medicine as they deemed necessary.

During the New Deal era, President Franklin Delano Roosevelt (FDR) planned for federally sponsored health insurance as part of the original Social Security Act of 1935. The country was facing a great depression, and FDR was tasked with helping improve the economy. During his first 100 days in office, FDR attempted to implement an unprecedented number of relief programs (Buck, 2017). Mention was made of a universal health program in the Social Security Bill, but information was not included in the bill or any recommendations about it. Instead, the Committee on Economic Security (CES) said it would make a later report about universal health insurance stating it needed more time to gather information. This innocent statement caused panic in the AMA thinking the federal government was secretly trying to pass compulsory health insurance onto the country without any details. Again, there was concern about federal involvement coming between physicians and their patients. Rumors spread and Americans became concerned, thus the universal health coverage was dropped before the signing of the Social Security Bill on August 14, 1935. What the Social Security Act of 1935 did was provide old age benefits, workman's compensation, unemployment insurance, and aid for dependent mothers and children, as well as the blind and physically handicapped (USA Facts, n.d.).

By this time, America was lagging on the world stage for national healthcare coverage. By the middle of the 1930s 25 countries in Europe, South America, and Asia had begun some form of national healthcare. President Harry S. Truman picked up where FDR left off stating, "the welfare and security of our nation demand the opportunity for good health be made available to all, regardless of residence, race or economic status" (National Archives, Harry S. Trumann. para 1). The US was in the middle of the Second World War and during this time there was a shift in thinking about state-run versus federally run programs. The US now had experience with programs such as old-age insurance and unemployment, plus the states were not doing as good a job of running them. In fact, the chaos created by these state-run programs prompted the Social Security Board to tell Congress that when recommending any national health insurance law, the states should be bypassed (Berkowitz, 2005–2006). Bills were introduced in 1943, 1945, and 1947 all featuring federal rather than state administration programs. "If any of these bills had passed health care would have been provided to all people of all ages" (Branyan & Peon, 1980).

By the 1950s, private insurance such as Blue Cross provided by employers had entered the scene. This underscored the need for public health insurance as these insurance companies became increasingly popular. Employees and their families could get insurance through their work as a benefit. It became clear that the deficits for health insurance were the elderly who were on social security and did not have a job, and the poor or disabled who were not working. In 1961, under President John F. Kennedy, the Medicare Bill began to receive attention. Emphasis was given to how passage of this bill would not undermine the authority or decisions of the physician or institution to allay fears that had been a previous issue (Berkowitz, 2005–2006). In 1965, after much debate and revision, Medicare, a federally run program for the elderly and Medicaid, a federally funded state-run program for the poor were signed into law. Thus, health insurance coverage was now available to the two most vulnerable populations: the old and the socially disadvantaged (see Figure 1.1).

UNDERSTANDING MEDICARE

As a nurse practitioner (NP), you may find the majority of reimbursement is paid by either Medicare or Medicaid. Private insurance plans follow the Medicare model, so understanding the essentials of Medicare will help you to obtain the care and services patients need. The following Medicare website helps patients navigate to a Medicare Advantage plan and drug benefits best suited for them: https://www.medicare.gov/plan-compare/#/?lang=en&year=2022

The beginning of the year is often the time when people make changes to their Medicare coverage. Medicare Part A applies primarily to inpatient hospital visits and for those who paid Medicare taxes, no premium is required (Medicare, n.d.). If a beneficiary is hospitalized, deductibles and co-pays may apply (CMS, 2022). Medicare Part B is optional and at low cost to the beneficiary, at $164.90 per month in 2023 (CMS, 2022). Medicare Part B covers primarily outpatient costs such as doctor office visits, labs, xrays, and outpatient surgery. Medicare Part B usually pays 80% with 20% costs as the

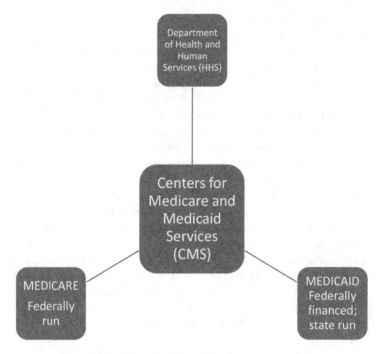

Figure 1.1 Hierarchy of Medicare and Medicaid programs

patient's responsibility. Medicare Parts A and B together are known as *Traditional Medicare* and beneficiaries have no in-network restrictions. A beneficiary of *Traditional Medicare* services can choose to purchase a supplemental policy to cover the 20% patient responsibility. Supplemental insurance can be costly yet choosing a Medicare Advangage plan (Part C) will have costs, coverage, and in-network requirements.

Medicare Advantage (MA or Part C) was signed into law by President Bill Clinton, in 1997. MA plans are managed healthcare plans run by health maintenance organizations (HMOs) and preferred provider organizations (PPOs). Under these plans, beneficiaries agree to the HMO or PPO terms (i.e., use in-network providers, obtain prior authorization for procedures) and pay no co-pay. Medicare Part C includes prescription drug coverage and other benefits including vision, dental, and hearing (KFF, 2021). The federal government pays MA plans a 10–15% administration fee as an incentive to keep costs low. The more money HMOs and PPOs save, the more money they keep (Schulte, 2023). There are mixed concerns with this profit driven incentive including inadequate treatment and denial of services.

MA plans, compared to *Traditional Medicare,* also have advantages and disadvantages. One advantage is, MA plans do what it is necessary to manage costs and decrease unnecessary services, making plans cost efficient. Yet, one disadvantage is the exact argument that the AMA put forth back in 1911 when sickness insurance was initially proposed: insurance plans, not the providers, are making care decisions. When patients, for example, are denied care or deemed ineligible for a test or skilled services, providers must write appeals to gain insurance approval. The MA business model seemed like a great idea until its implementation created barriers to care and services. Despite this problem, MA plans have grown in popularity in part by the heavy marketing of drug coverage, dental care, and vision services – prior to Medicare Part D, MA plans were and still are inticing.

On December 8, 2003, President George W. Bush signed into law Medicare Part D. Medicare Part D offers prescription drug coverage and there are multiple options with varying costs (see Figure 1.2).

Medicare Part D can be confusing for patients and providers however it is important that the NP understands Medicare Part D, specifically medication costs because costs will directly impact whether the patient can afford a prescribed medication. In 2020, the average retiree's social security income (SSI) was $1478 a month (KFF, n.d.). Some medications can be cost prohibitive for patients living on SSI income.

Initially, Part D paid for a number of medicines with a small copay. Yet, when the beneficiary fell into a *donut hole* they were responsible for 100% of the pharmacy bill up to $2000. The donut hole created a scenario where seniors found themselves going from an affordable monthly bill for medications to paying full price. Providers scrambled for workarounds to provide their patients with medications including substituing generic medication or providing sample medications.

To fix this problem the rules changed in 2019 when President Donald Trump signed the Bipartisan Budget Act of 2018. In 2022, beneficiaries pay an initial deductable of $480 and then they have a co-pay for about 25% of the bill which can still be significant if they are on medications which are expensive. Below are the current terms of Medicare Part D (see Tables 1.1–1.4).

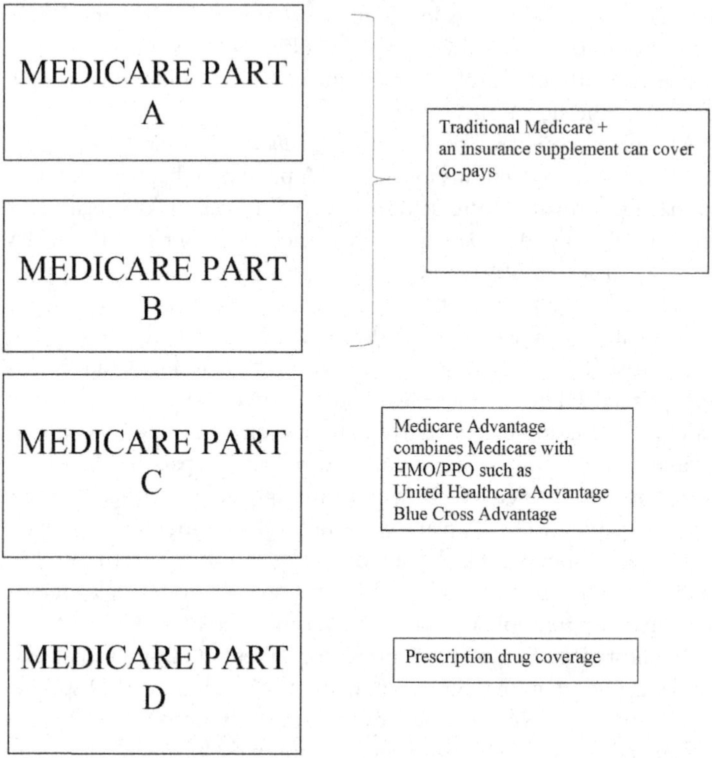

Figure 1.2 Overview of Medicare Part D

Table 1.1 Breakdown of Part D Coverage

Deductible	Patient responsibility – $480		
Initial phase up to $4430	*75% plan covers cost of medication*	*25% patient responsibility*	
Gap phase up to $7050	*70% DISCOUNT from manufacturer*	*5% plan pays*	*25% patient responsibility*
Catastrophic phase after $7050 has been spent	*80% Medicare pays*	*15% plan pays*	*5% patient responsibility*

Table 1.2 shows an example with Medicare Part D and two medications:

Patient pays the first $480.

Table 1.2 Coverage up to initial $4430

Drug name	Retail cost	Plan pays	Patient pays
Breo inhaler	$464	$348	$116
Spiriva Respimat	$576	$432	$144
			$260 monthly

Table 1.3 Coverage gap phase up to $7050

Drug name	Retail cost	Discount by manufacturer	Plan pays	Patient pays
Breo	$464	$324	$23.00	$117.00
Spiriva	$576	$403	$28.80	$144.20
				$261.20 monthly

Table 1.4 Catastrophic coverage phase with brand name

Drug name	Retail cost	Medicare pays	Plan pays	Patient pays
Breo	$464	$371	$70	*9.95 is lessor amount*
Spiriva	$576	$461	$86	*9.95 is lessor amount*
				$19.90 a month

As a NP being mindful of prescription costs and the patient's ability to pay are essential to manage your Medicare patients. Look for generic medications whenever you can and remember that coupons provided by drug representatives **DO NOT** cover name-brand drugs when the insurance source is Medicare or Medicaid. The reason coupons do not work for this category is because Medicare and Medicaid Part D plans have already negotiated a lower price for the medications with the drug companies.

You can also see why Part D plans during the initial phase avoid covering brand name medications and require generics to be utilized first because brand name medications cost more for the insurance plans to cover during that phase (KFF, 2021 October 13).

Finally, in 2010 President Barack Obama signed into law the Affordable Care Act (ACA) with the intention of making insurance accessible and affordable for all people and bringing US citizens closer to the goal of having national health insurance. However, the roll out of the ACA did not go as smoothly as planned and legislators on both sides of the aisle are looking for ways to improve the ACA, so that someday the US may have affordable healthcare for all Americans.

THE BUSINESS OF HEALTHCARE

Healthcare is a business that has two sides: the patient side and the business side. One hundred years ago a medical encounter was a transaction between a physician and a patient through the exchange of money or in the form of bartering for services. Many physicians were paid for their services in eggs or other commodities. In 1929, the medium income for a physician in the US was $3758 annually (Weinfeld, 1951). It was argued that health insurance would provide a steady income to physicians to allieviate this problem, but as mentioned before the AMA was opposed to nationalizing health insurance because they did not want the government to interfere between the physician and patient care decisions. However, with the passage of Medicare and Medicaid in 1965, reimbursement for services to providers and hospitals was solidly pumped into the system, raising doctors' income into the upper-middle-class tier and beyond (Berkowitz, 2005–2006). Providers were pleased with the fact that the government kept its promise and did not meddle between the physician and patient care. This environment created a booming healthcare industry. Investment was made in medical schools to produce more providers and research to combat disease. Physicians no longer worried about reimbursement and could practice medicine the way they saw fit.

Healthcare services for the young and old were primarily billed to Medicare and Medicaid. Increased services created an increase in billing and the need for accountability. To standardize and manage the billing process, Congress established the evaluation and management (E/M) standards and guidelines for Medicare, which were published originally in 1995. Revisions were made in 1997, 2021, and most recently the newest revisions became effective on January 1, 2023. These rules provide a standard guideline to determine the type and severity of patient conditions, so that reimbursement for services can be expedited in an organized and timely way. This fee schedule was adopted by private health insurance companies as the standard to follow.

As NPs, documentation is required for several reasons. One reason to record the NP and patient encounter is so that the NP can review what was done and why. The other reason is to justify the payment of a bill by showing services utilized and reasons why. E/M rules provide a structure for NPs to document what they did, and the clinical reasoning with each encounter, so that when the bill is submitted to the insurance company, the level of care billed is supported. The process is straightforward and once you are famililar with each step and the rules, it becomes easy to capture payment for the services rendered.

A practice can not survive without adequate revenue, which is the business side. As much as NPs would like to provide services to all people without the worry of expense, the reality is, a practice will have limited finances for expenses. To buy new equipment, better equipment, or hire more people requires income. Accurate E/M documentation of the NP–patient encounter based on the time and services provided can help supply income for running a practice. Billing for *more* or *less* than what is appropriate with Medicare or Medicaid however, is not acceptable and can result in fines, loss of licensure, and or prison.

Here is an example of one medical practice's monthly set expenses.

SAMPLE PRACTICE EXPENSES

Advertising	$500
Insurance	$2000
Office supplies	$1000
EMR and billing software	$450
Wages and benefits for employees	$25000 (one provider plus 2 medical assistants and a front office person)
Taxes	$2000
Telephone	$500
Rent	$4000
Total	**$35,450**

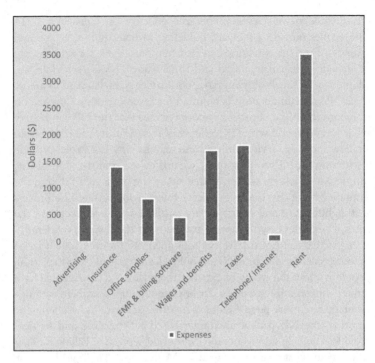

Figure 1.3 Example medical practice expenses

Below is an example of billing codes from the American Medical Association (AMA) physican fee schedule for 2022 for an established patient in an office environment such as the practice above. Notice the *lower amount* of reimbursement for the NP visit compared to the physician reimbursement. In 1997, when the Balanced Budget Act passed, NPs could bill Medicare directly for services. However, that reimbursement rate was set at 85% of a physician's rate (Bischof & Greenberg, 2021). The physician versus NP reimbursement rate has been a topic of debate by professional NP associations. Note the work relative value units (wRVU) in the last column, an important value that will be discussed in this section.

Now use the following chart and figure out how many patients your practice would need to see daily in each category to make your bottom line of $35,420 dollars in monthly expenses.

Table 1.5 Example of billing codes for an established patient visiting a practice

Established patient office visit	Physician reimbursement ($)	NP reimbursement ($)	wRVU
99211	23.53	20.00	0.18
99212	57.45	48.83	0.70
99213	92.05	78.24	1.30
99214	129.77	110.30	1.92
99215	183.07	155.60	2.80

Table 1.6 Template for calculating number of patients needed to meet monthly expenses

Established patient office visit	#	NP reimbursement ($)	Total ($)	wRVU
99211		20.00		0.18
99212		48.83		0.70
99213		78.24		1.30
99214		110.30		1.92
99215		155.60		2.80

If you found that you needed to see patients mainly in the 99213 to 99215 range, you would be correct. If you also found you would need to see between 20 and 25 patients a day to meet your expenses you would also be right. You could hire another provider to help with the workload, but this would raise your practice expenses and you would have to adjust accordingly. As you can see from this activity the documentation captured for your services for correct billing can make or break your practice.

WHAT ARE wRVUs?

Work relative value units (wRVUs) are important to undestand in negotiating your contracts. Many of you have signed agreements that state how many wRVUs you are required to attain and once you do, what a bonus structure will look like. The more wRVUs you generate the more valuable you are to the team because it equates to how much revenue you can generate for the practice. Let's take a minute to understand what wRVUs are.

The Social Security Act of 1992 requires the Centers for Medicare and Medicaid Services (CMS) to establish payment based on a national uniform *relative value unit*. These units of measurement have become known as RVUs. RVUs take into consideration the following 3 factors: physician work, geographic practice cost indicies, and practice expenses including malpractice in the following formula: [physician work (wRVU) ★ the geographic practice cost indicies (GPCI)] + [physician expense (PE) ★ the GPCI], + [malpractice (MP) ★ GPCI] x conversion factor based on different specialties and demographics. This formula is complicated and you do not need memorize it, but it is helpful for you to see that if your practice is located in a high cost of living area, or is a specialty with high malpractice insurance, reimbursement takes into account these factors to create a *level playing field for all providers*. Let's follow a bill and see how RVUs play into the reimbursement rate.

ROUTE TAKEN BY A BILL

1. A patient chart is coded with a CPT (current procedural terminology) number for level of service provided (your documentation supports this).
2. Your practice sends Medicare or a private insurer the bill.
3. Medicare looks at the CPT codes (justifies it by your documentation if audited) and assigns a relative value unit (RVU) to each of them.
4. Medicare enters the wRVUs for the patient visit into a conversion factor (CF) equation to get the dollar amount for the reimbursement to your practice.
5. Medicare sends you a check for your services.

Conversion formula: (wRVU x GPCI) + (PE RVU x GPCI) + (MP RVU x GPCI) x CF = payment (Chaplain, 2021).

Table 1.7 Conversion formula for a practice in two separate locations

wRVU x w GPCI	PE RVU x PE GPCI	MPRVU x MPGPCI	Total RVUs x CF	
East St. Louis				
9.49 * 0.986 +	10.71 PE *.942 +	1.9 MP * 1.661 =	22.600 * (32.00)	$723.20
Long Island				
9.49 * 1.046 +	10.71 * 1.223 +	1.9 * 2.702 =	28.158 * (32.00)	$901.00

Source: (American Academy of Professional Coders [AAPC], n.d.)

The example given in Table 1.7 uses two distinct locations but the *same* procedure.

You can see the practice in Long Island got paid $177.80 more than the practice in East St. Louis for the *exact* same procedure. This is because Medicare makes adjustments based on costs associated with practice expenses, geographic area, and specialty malpractice insurance and reimburses at a fair and equitable rate for each location.

REFERENCES

American Academy of Professional Coders. (n.d.). *What are relative value units (RVUs)?* AAPC. Retrieved from https://www.aapc.com/practice-management/rvus.aspx"https://www.aapc.com/practice-management/rvus.aspx

Berkowitz, E. (2005–2006). Medicare and Medicaid: The past as prologue. *Health Care Finance Rev, 27*(2), 11–23. https://pubmed.ncbi.nlm.nih.gov/17290633/

Bischof, A. & Greenberg, S. (2021). Post Covid-19 reimbursement parity for nurse practitioners. *The Online Journal of Issues in Nursing, 26*(2).

Branyan, R. L. & Peon, M. (1980). Harry S. Truman versus the medical lobby: The genesis of Medicare. *The Journal of American History, 66*(4), 983. https://doi.org/10.2307/1887731

Buck, S. (2017, June 15). *Universal health care was almost part of the original Social Security Act of 1935.* Timeline. Retrieved February 24, 2022, from https://timeline.com/social-security-universal-health-care-efe875bbda93

Chaplain, S. (2021, November 1). *Relative value units: The basis of medicare payments.* AAPC Knowledge Center. https://www.aapc.com/blog/82531-relative-value-units-the-basis-of-medicare-payments-2/#:~:text=Here%-E2%80%99s%20the%20complete%20formula%20used%20to%20arrive%20at,x%20MP%20GPCI%29%5D%20x%20CF%20%3D%20final%20payment

CMS (2022). 2023 Medicare Parts A & B premiums and deductibles 2023 Medicare Part D income-related monthly adjustment amounts. Retrieved from https://www.cms.gov/newsroom/fact-sheets/2023-medicare-parts-b-premiums-and-deductibles-2023-medicare-part-d-income-related-monthly

Hirshfield, D. (1970). *The campaign for compulsory health insurance in the United States from 1932 to 1943*. Harvard University Press, Cambridge, MA.

KFF. (2021). Payments to Medicare Advantage plans boosted the Medicare spending by $7 billion in 2019. Retrieved from https://www.kff.org/medicare/press-release/payments-to-medicare-advantage-plans-boosted-medicare-spending-by-7-billion-in-2019/

KFF. (2021, October 13). *An overview of the Medicare Part D prescription drug benefit*. Retrieved from https://www.kff.org/medicare/fact-sheet/an-overview-of-the-medicare-part-d-prescription-drug-benefit/"https://www.kff.org/medicare/fact-sheet/an-overview-of-the-medicare-part-d-prescription-drug-benefit/

Medicare (n.d.). 2023 Medicare costs. Retrieved from https://www.medicare.gov/Pubs/pdf/11579-medicare-costs.pdf

National Archives. Harry S. Truman. Special Message to the Congress on Health and Disability Insurance, para 1. https://www.trumanlibrary.gov/library/public-papers/98/special-message-congress-health-and-disability-insurance

Rubinow, I. (1916). *Social insurance with special reference to American conditions*. Henry Holt and Company, New York City, NY.

Schulte, F. (2023) Government lets health plans that ripped off Medicare keep the money. KHN. Retrieved from https://khn.org/news/article/cms-audits-medicare-advantage-plans-can-keep-hundreds-of-millions-in-federal-overpayments-maybe-more/

USA Facts. (n.d.). *Social security average retirement monthly benefit*. Retrieved February 23, 2022, from https://usafacts.org/data/topics/people-society/social-security-and-medicare/social-security/social-security-average-monthly-benefit/?utm_source=bing&utm_medium=cpc&utm_campaign=ND-StatsData&msclkid=cf0e5165c18e14584aa0308535955340

Weinfeld, W. (1951, July). *Income of physicians, 1929–49* [PDF]. https://fraser.stlouisfed.org/files/docs/publications/SCB/pages/1950-1954/4374_1950-1954.pdf

GENERAL PRINCIPLES OF MEDICAL RECORD DOCUMENTATION

E/M visits are categorized by the location of the service that has taken place or been provided. Within each of these categories are 3–5 subcategories related to the level of service provided. E/M codes **ALWAYS** begin with the digit **"99"**.

SUBCATEGORIES RELATED TO SERVICE LEVEL

TYPE OF PATIENT

- **New patient** – per the AMA CPT guidelines pg 6 para 5 *"a new patient is one who has not received any professional services from the physician/qualified healthcare professional or another physician/qualified healthcare professional of the exact same specialty and subspecialty who belongs to the same group practice, **within the past three years.**"*
- **Established patient** – per the AMA CPT guidelines pg 6 para 6 *"one who has received professional services from the physician/qualified healthcare professional or another physician/qualified healthcare professional of the exact same specialty and subspecialty who belongs to the same group practice **within the past three years.**"*

(See Figure 2.1.)

DOI: 10.4324/9781003542872-2

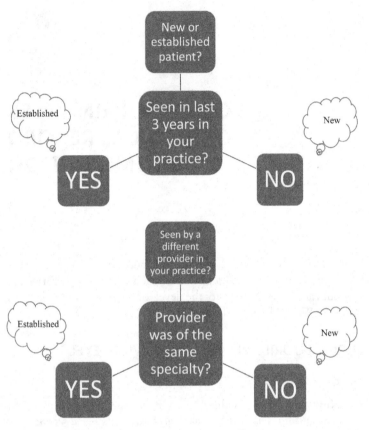

Figure 2.1 Decision tree for new and established patients

Source: AMA 2022

TYPE OF SERVICE

- New or established office/outpatient visit
- Hospital services/ER services
- Consultation services
- Nursing facility services, domiciliary, rest home, or custodial care services
- Home services
- Telehealth services

LEVEL OF SERVICE (PER 2023 GUIDELINES)

- Straightforward
- Low risk
- Medium risk

COMMON TTRMS

- **Qualified healthcare professional:** a qualified individual by education and training or licensure who performs a professional service within their scope of practice.
- **Professional service:** a face-to-face service provided by a physician or a qualified healthcare professional.
- **Clinical staff member:** a person who works under the direction of a physician or qualified healthcare professional.

DEFINITIONS FROM THE AMA (HOLLMANN ET AL., N.D.)

- **Self-limited or minor problem:** a problem that runs a definite and prescribed course, is transient in nature, and is not likely to permanently alter health status.
- **Stable, chronic illness:** duration of at least a year until the death of the patient.
- **Acute, uncomplicated illness or injury:** recent or new short-term problem with minimal risk of morbidity for which treatment is considered. There is little to no risk of mortality with treatment and full recovery without functional impairment is expected.

LET'S PRACTICE: NEW OR ESTABLISHED PATIENT?*

EXERCISE 1

Encounter 1: MJ was seen 1/1/2000 by Dr. Smith an internal medicine doctor.
Encounter 2: MJ has been seen 1/1/2001 by the NP in the same practice.
Encounter 3: MJ is now seen by Dr. Smith 1/1/2003.

EXERCISE 2

Encounter 1: RG was seen by Dr. Owen on 1/2/2003 to establish care with primary care.

Encounter 2: RG saw Dr. Clarence a cardiologist on 2/10/2004 who is in the same office with the same practice.

Encounter 3: RG comes back to see Dr. Owens NP on 1/30/2006.

*Answers at the end of the chapter.

In the case of a NP covering a call for another provider, the billing code should be the same as if the *original provider* saw the patient. For example, if you had an internal medicine provider from another practice covering for your family practice clinic one day the covering provider would bill patients as if they were being seen at your practice. Thus even though the patients are new to the on-call NP of another practice, they are established with your practice.

INTERNATIONAL CLASSIFICATION OF DISEASES (ICD) CODES VERSES CPT CODES

The purpose of the international code of diseases (ICD) was to track causes of death within populations. The development of these codes can be traced back to 1763 to a French physician, Dr. Francois Bossier de Sauvages de Lacroix when he developed 10 disease classifications. These 10 diseases were further subdivided into 2400 unique diseases. This led to the need for an international list to be created that could be utilized by all nations. The first International Statistical Congress was held in 1853.

In 1948, the World Health Organization was charged with maintaining this list and expanded it to include mortality and morbidity. Currently, the ICD-10th edition was implemented on October 1, 2015, and includes more detail and specificity on disease codes than the previous edition. ICD codes are important for payment by all payers. First, ICD codes provide a *diagnosis code*. Secondly, if tests are ordered they are linked to the correct ICD code that justifies ordering the test. ICD codes are updated every decade (Hirsch et al., 2016).

Examples of ICD-10 codes:

H65.19 Acute Otitis Media
J03.00 Strep Throat
N39.0 Urinary Tract Infection
J12.82 Covid 19
E03.9 Hypothyroidism

CPT CODES

Current Procedural Terminology coding system (CPT) is published by the AMA with the assistance of the Centers for Medicare and Medicaid Services (CMS). Initially in the mid1960s, the AMA worked with multiple medical specialties and developed a coding system that would describe medical services and procedures billed. The very first CPT book was released in 1966 and contained only surgical codes. Since that time, the CPT codes have expanded and now include all the tests or procedures you may do during an office visit.

Examples of CPT *procedural* codes:

CPT 69209   Cerumen impaction removal
CPT 85025   CBC
CPT 84443   TSH

To get paid for a procedure the NP must link the correct disease code (ICD) to the correct procedure code (CPT). In the following example you can see why this would be denied payment because a diagnosis of strep throat would not necessitate the removal of cerumen. ICD J03.00 strep throat **does not go with** CPT 69209 cerumen impaction removal. However, suppose the patient did have strep throat and during the examination, you found a cerumen impaction and took care of it. You would correctly link the ICD code for cerumen impaction to the CPT code of cerumen impaction removal, and the ICD code for strep throat with the CPT code rapid strep test and you would get reimbursed for your services.

H61.21 Cerumen impaction **goes with** CPT 69209 Cerumen impaction removal.

J03.00 Strep Throat **goes with** CPT 87880 Rapid Group A Strep antigen.

This applies to all procedures for example skin biopsies, stitches, incision and drainage, strep testing, flu testing, lab work, radiological imaging, or joint injections. They are all examples of *procedural* CPT codes that would need to be linked to the correct ICD code for payment to be made.

Initially, CPT codes did not have a relationship with reimbursement for the actual visit, but over time this has changed. With the implementation of the Health Insurance Portability and Accountability Act (HIPAA) CPT codes were expanded beyond procedural service reporting and facilitated a way to report and be reimbursed for services in a fee for service model (Hirsch et al., 2016).

E/M codes are a category of CPT codes used for billing purposes and represent the level of care and complexity of that patient visit or encounter. E/M coding is at the heart of every medical practice and understanding the documentation process is crucial for any provider billing for services.

Review the following bill submitted to Medicare for reimbursement for the level of service (office visit) and testing ordered.

E/M SERVICES

E/M guidelines support the evaluation and management of the patient. As discussed, earlier E/Ms were developed by the AMA in conjunction with the CMS. They are a subset of CPT codes. The first set was released in 1995, and the second set was released in 1997. It was up to the provider to decide which set of rules to follow for billing their services, but they could only follow one set or the other; they could not combine the two. Both the 1995 and 1997 E/M guidelines were built upon the documentation of three **building blocks** (History, Physical Exam, and Medical Decision

Table 2.1 Bill detailing appropriate service and procedure codes

Bill	Criteria	Payment
CPT 99204 **Level of service code**	*Documentation supports this level of service*	*Approved*
CPT 8443 (TSH- thyroid stimulating hormone test) **Procedural code**	*ICDE03.9 – Hypothyroidism diagnosis*	*Approved*

Making) in the encounter and within those blocks were subcomponents that also had requirements. There were documentation rules for what type of history of present illness (HPI) a provider needed to document such as brief or extensive, as well as how many elements of past family social history (PFSH) or review of systems (ROS), and what type of physical exam was needed to be performed for each level, and finally the medical decision-making tool. Notice the 1995 rules differ from the 1997 rules **ONLY in the physical exam** component of the equation, everything else stayed the same. In the 1995 rules, the physical exam consisted of choosing between 12 organ systems or 7 body areas to document with *limited direction*. Providers and insurance auditors did not have a clear distinction between *limited* or *extended.* This led to wide speculation and adjustments to submitted bills depending on the auditor's point of view. The 1997 rules attempted to correct this by further dividing the **body systems/areas into 14** and adding **specific bullet points** that must be documented to get credit but as Figure 2.2 shows it may have been **TOO** specific and added to the confusion.

Because of the excessive burden of documentation, changes to the E/M guidelines were updated on January 1, 2021, for **office and outpatient visits only**, as a pilot. The workgroup established to devise these changes was charged with simplifying the work of the healthcare provider while improving the health of the patient. They had four guiding principles:

1. Decrease administrative burden.
2. Decrease the need for audits.

3.   Decrease unnecessary documentation.
4.   Ensure payment for the E/M is resource based.

HISTORY *			
Chief Complaint			
	HPI	**PFSH**	**ROS**
Problem focused	Brief (1–3)	None	None
EPF	Brief (1–3)	None	1
Detailed	EXT (4 or more)	1 of 3	2–9
Comprehensive	Ext (4 or more or 3 chronic conditions)	3 of 3 (Except in ER 2/3)	10
PHYSICAL EXAM			
		1995 Rules	**1997 Rules**
Problem focused		A limited exam of the affected body areas or organ system (at least 1)	1–5 exam bullets
Extended problem focused		A **limited exam** of the affected body area or organ system and other symptomatic or related organ system(s)	6–11 exam bullets
Detailed		An **extended exam** of the affected body area and other symptomatic or related organ system(s)	12 exam bullets
Comprehensive		A general multi-system examination or complete examination of a single organ system* (8–12 organ system)	2 bullets from NINE systems
MEDICAL DECISION MAKING *			
MDM level	**Problem points**	**Data points**	**Risk**
Straightforward	≤1	≤1	Minimal
Low	2	2	Low
Moderate	3	3	Moderate
High	≥4	≥4	High
Calculate the level to be billed: • Level of Care for **History**_____ • Level of Care for **Physical exam**_____ • Level of Care for **Medical decision making**_____			

*History and MDM level best 2 out of 3

Figure 2.2 E/M Worksheet 1995/1997 rules

No longer would documentation be based on the 3 building blocks of History, Physical Exam (PE), and Medical Decision Making (MDM). From this point, the provider would document an ***appropriate history and physical exam***. Billing and coding would be based only on the MDM or time; whichever was longer.

Table 2.2 1995 Physical exam requirements (no directions on what to document)

12 Organ systems	7 Body areas
Constitutional	Head, including face
Eyes	Neck
ENMT	Chest, including breasts/axillae
Cardiovascular	Abdomen
Respiratory	Genitalia, groin, buttocks
Gastrointestinal	Back, including spine
Genitourinary	
Musculoskeletal	
Skin	
Neurologic	
Psychiatric	
Hematologic/Lymph/Immune	

Source: 1995 AMA E/M guidelines

ANSWERS TO EXERCISES

Exercise 1:

Encounter 1: Bill as New to practice.

Encounter 2: Bill as Established patient as seen by equivalent provider in same practice.

Encounter 3: Bill as Established patient because patient has been seen by equivalent provider in same practice within 3 years.

Exercise 2:

Encounter 1: Bill as NEW patient as patient is new to practice of internal medicine.

Encounter 2: Bill as NEW patient as cardiologist may be in the same practice but is not of the same specialty.

Encounter 3: Bill as NEW patient because he has not been seen by primary care within 3 years.

Table 2.3 1997 Physical exam rules (too much direction on what to document)

Systems/body area	Elements of examination
Constitutional	• Measurement of any three of the following seven vital signs: Sitting or standing BP (blood pressure), supine blood pressure, pulse rate and regularity, respiration, temp, height, weight (may be measured and recorded by ancillary staff) • General appearance of patient
Eyes	• Inspection of conjunctivae and lids • Examination of pupils and irises (reaction to light and accommodation, size, and symmetry) • Ophthalmoscopic examination of optic discs
Ears, Nose, Mouth and Throat	• External inspection of ears and nose • Otoscopic examination of external auditory canals and TM • Assessment of hearing • Inspection of nasal mucosa, septum, and turbinates • Inspection of lips, teeth, and gums • Examination of oropharynx
Neck	• Examination of neck (eg, masses, overall appearance, symmetry, tracheal position, crepitus) • Examination of thyroid (eg, enlargement, tenderness, mass)
Respiratory	• Assessment of respiratory effort • Percussion of chest • Palpation of chest • Auscultation of lungs
Cardiovascular	• Palpation of heart • Auscultation of heart with notation of abnormal sounds and murmurs • Examination of:

Table 2.3 1997 (Continued)

Systems/body area	Elements of examination
	• *Carotid arteries* • *Abdominal aorta* • *Femoral arteries* • *Pedal pulses* • *Extremities for edema and or varicosities*
Chest (breast)	• *Inspection of breasts* • *Palpation of breasts and axillae*
Gastrointestinal (abdomen)	• *Examination of abdomen with notation of presence of masses or tenderness* • *Examination of liver and spleen* • *Examination for presence or absence of hernia* • *Examination (when indicated) of anus, perineum, and rectum, including sphincter tone, presence of hemorrhoids, rectal masses* • *Obtain stool sample for occult blood test when indicated*
Genitourinary	*MALE* • *Examination of the scrotal contents* • *Examination of the penis* • *Digital rectal exam of prostate gland* *FEMALE* *Pelvic examination (with or without specimen collection for smears and cultures), including* • *Examination of external genitalia* • *Examination of urethra* • *Examination of bladder* • *Cervix* • *Uterus* • *Adnexa/parametria*
Lymphatic	*Palpation of lymph nodes in two or more areas* • *Neck* • *Axillae* • *Groin* • *Other*

(Continued)

Table 2.3 1997 (Continued)

Systems/body area	Elements of examination
Musculoskeletal	• *Examination of gait and station* • *Inspection and or palpation of digits and nails* *Examination of joints, bones, and muscles of one or more of the following six areas: head and neck; spine, ribs, and* *pelvis, right upper extremity, left upper extremity, right lower extremity and left lower extremity. The examination of a given area includes:ç* • *Inspection and or palpation with notation of presence of any misalignment, asymmetry, crepitation, defects, tenderness, masses, effusions* • *Assessment of range of motion with notation of any pain, crepitation, or contracture* • *Assessment of stability with notation of any dislocation (luxation), subluxation or laxity* • *Assessment of muscle strength and tone (eg, flaccid, cog wheel, spastic with notation of any atrophy or abnormal movements*
Skin	*Inspection of skin and subcutaneous tissue (eg, rashes, lesions, ulcers)* • *Palpation of skin and subcutaneous tissue (eg, induration, subcutaneous nodules, tightening)*
Neurological	*Test cranial nerves with notation of any deficits.* • *Examination of deep tendon reflexes with notation of pathological reflexes (eg. Babinski)* • *Examination of sensation (eg, by touch, pin, vibration, proprioception)*
Psychiatric	• *Description of patient's judgment and insight* • *Brief assessment of mental status including:* • *Orientation to time, place, and person* • *Recent and remote memory* • *Mood and affect (eg, depression, anxiety, agitation)*

Source: 1997 AMA E/M guidelines

REFERENCES

American Medical Association. (2022). *CPT 2022 Professional Edition.* American Medical Association.

Centers for Medicare and Medicaid. (n.d.-a). *1995 Documentation guidelines for evaluation and management services.* https://www.cms.gov/Outreach-and-Education/Medicare-Learning-Network-MLN/MLNEdWebGuide/Downloads/95Docguidelines.pdf

Centers for Medicare and Medicaid. (n.d.-b). *1997 Documentation guidelines for evaluation and management services.* Retrieved February 23, 2022, from https://www.cms.gov/Outreach-and-Education/Medicare-Learning-Network-MLN/MLNEdWebGuide/Downloads/97Docguidelines.pdf

Hirsch, J., Nicola, G., McGinty, G., Liu, R., Barr, R., Chittle, M., & Manchikanti, L. (2016). ICD-10: History and context. *American Journal of Neuroradiology, 37*(4), 596–599. https://doi.org/10.3174/ajnr.a4696

Hollmann, P., MD, Jagmin, C., MD, & Levy, B., MD. (n.d.). *Evaluation and management (E/M) office visits – 2021.* American Medical Association. Retrieved February 23, 2022, from https://www.ama-assn.org/system/files/2020-04/e-m-office-visit-changes.pdf

DOCUMENTATION

Documentation as a NP is important for the following reasons:

- To record every patient encounter describing the subjective and objective data, physical exam findings, treatment plan, and patient education.
- To communicate to all members of the healthcare team the plan for patient care.
- To determine the correct coding and billing for reimbursement of services.

The most recent 2023 E/M coding changes related to documentation are that the providers no longer need to document a certain number of history and physical exam elements. Instead, coding and billing are assessed by the provider's documentation of medical decision making (MDM) or time whichever yields the better reimbursement. This means it is still important to document the necessary history and physical examination of the patient encounter; however, it is vital to document your process of medical decision making. The MDM tool has been revised and is comprised of the following 3 elements.

1. Number and **C**omplexity **O**f **P**roblems **A**ddressed during the patient encounter **(COPA)**

DOI: 10.4324/9781003542872-3

2. Amount and complexity of **DATA** to be reviewed or analyzed (DATA)
3. **RISK** of complications and/or morbidity or mortality of patient management (RISK)

These three elements of MDM determine the E/M visit code for billing based on the level of complexity of the patient encounter. Levels of complexity are straightforward, low, moderate, or high complexity. Using the following table, read the example documentation of a visit with subsequent billing.

DOCUMENTATION EXAMPLE

The NP is caring for Mr. Smith for the first patient visit. He is obese and has poorly controlled hypertension. His BP today is 160/98. He is unemployed and only takes his antihypertensive medications sporadically because he can't afford his medications and has no transportation to the pharmacy. During your visit, you take a history and perform a complete medical examination, order a CMP, CBC and A1C to assess any comorbid conditions such as impaired renal function, anemias and diabetes mellitus type 2 and change his antihypertensive medications to generics to reduce the cost to the patient. You provide resources for the patient to receive his medications by delivery or mail.

- **Element 1** – Number of problems: the patient has obesity and poorly controlled hypertension. (Moderate)
- **Element 2** – Complexity Of Data Reviewed: The NP ordered a CBC, CBC, and AIC and assessed his BP. (Low)
- **Element 3** – Risk of Complications and or Morbidity: The NP changed his antihypertensive medications considering his social and economic barriers. (Moderate)

Using the following chart and assuming this was an office visit of an established patient, the code would be 99214 unless time was the deciding factor.

Table 3.1 2023 MDM tool

MDM (Based on 2 out of 3 elements of MDM)	COPA	DATA	RISK
99211	*N/A*	*N/A*	*N/A*
Straightforward 99202 99212 99221 99231 99234	*1 self-limited or minor problem*	*Minimal or NONE*	*Minimal risk of morbidity from additional diagnostic testing or treatment*
Low complexity 99203 99213 99221 99231 99234	*2 or more self-limited or minor problems* **or** *1 stable, chronic illness* **or** *1 acute uncomplicated illness or injury* **or** *1 stable, acute illness*	*(Must meet 1 of 2 requirements)* **Category 1: Tests and documents** *Any combination of 2 from the following* • *Review of prior external note(s) from each unique source* • *Review of the result(s) of each unique test* • *Ordering of each unique test*	*Low risk of morbidity from additional diagnostic testing or treatment*
	or *1 acute, uncomplicated illness or injury requiring hospital inpatient or observation level of care*	*OR* **Category 2: Assessment requiring an independent historian(s)**	

(Continued)

Table 3.1 (Continud)

Moderate	1 or more chronic illnesses with exacerbation, progression, or side effects of treatment	(Must meet requirements 1 out of 3)	Moderate risk of morbidity from additional diagnostic testing or treatment
99204 99214 99222 99232 99235		**Category 1: Tests, documents, historian**	Examples only:
	or 2 or more stable chronic illnesses	Any combination of 3 from the following	• *Prescription drug management*
	or 1 undiagnosed new problem with uncertain prognosis	• Review of prior external note(s) from each unique source	• *Decision regarding minor surgery with identified patient or procedure risk factors*
	or 1 acute illness with systemic symptoms	• Review of the result(s) of each unique test • Ordering of each unique test	• *Decision regarding elective major surgery without identified patient or procedure risk factors.*
	or 1 acute, complicated injury	• Assessment requiring an independent historian(s)	
		or **Category 2: Independent interpretation of tests**	
		• Independent interpretation of a test performed by another physician/ other qualified healthcare professional (not separately reported)	

Table 3.1 (Continud)

		or **Category 3: Discussion of management or test interpretation.**	• *Diagnosis or treatment significantly limited by social determinants of health*
		• *Discussion of management or test interpretation with external/ physician/ other qualified healthcare professional/ appropriate source (not separately reported)*	
High complexity 99205 99215 99223 99233 99236	*1 or more chronic illnesses with severe exacerbation, progression, or side effects of treatment* **or** *1 acute or chronic illness or injury that poses a threat to life or bodily function* **or** *Multiple morbidities requiring intensive management (Initial Nursing Facility only)*	*(Must meet 2 out of 3 requirements)* **Category 1: Tests, documents, historian** *Any combination of 3 from the following* • *Review of prior external note(s) from each unique source* • *Review of the result(s) of each unique test* • *Ordering of each unique test* • *Assessment requiring an independent historian(s)*	*High risk of morbidity from additional diagnostic testing or treatment* Examples only: • *Drug therapy requiring intensive monitoring for toxicity* • *Decision for elective major surgery with identified patient or procedure risk factors*

(Continued)

Table 3.1 (Continud)

---

or

Category 2: Independent interpretation of tests

- *Independent interpretation of a test performed by another physician/ other qualified healthcare professional (not separately reported)*

or

Category 3: Discussion of management or test interpretation

- *Discussion of management or test interpretation with external/ physician/ other qualified healthcare professional/ appropriate source (not separately reported)*

- *Decision for emergency major surgery*
- *Decision regarding hospitalization*
- *Decision for DNR or to de-escalate care because of poor prognosis*
- *Parenteral controlled substances*

E/M CODING USING TIME

Documentation can now be based on time only if that increases your level of complexity. When documenting time, it is important to state the time spent and what was performed. This needs to be accurate and not exaggerated. For example, *"During this patient visit today, 45 mins was spent on reviewing previous patient encounters regarding his hypertension and pre-diabetes. I reviewed previous patient notes, lab tests, and direct patient care today discussing the status of his poorly controlled hypertension and gave him resources to get patient assistance for medication and pharmacy delivery."*

TYPES OF DOCUMENTATION

There are different types of documentation for different purposes. For example, you may be documenting a well visit (adult or child), a chronic or acute care management visit versus a Medicare wellness visit. Each type of visit requires a different type of documentation to be medically appropriate as follows.

PREVENTIVE MEDICAL SERVICES (WELL VISITS)

Preventive services or wellness visits are continued throughout the lifespan. If during the examination, you find a problem that requires additional work up you would report a normal office visit code with modifier 25 and code the preventive service separately. However, if the problem is minor and does not require additional work up you would proceed with the normal preventive service code.

Table 3.2 New comprehensive preventive medicine

99381	*Age younger than 1 year*
99382	*Age 1–4*
99383	*Age 5–11*
99384	*Age 12–17*
99385	*Age 18–39*
99386	*Age 40–64*
99387	*Age 65 and older* **(MEDICARE DOES NOT PAY FOR THIS)**

Table 3.3 Established periodic patient preventive medicine

99391	*Age younger than 1 year*
99392	*Age 1–4*
99393	*Age 5–11*
99394	*Age 12–17*
99395	*Age 18–39*
99396	*Age 40–64*
99397	*Age 65 and older* **(MEDICARE DOES NOT PAY FOR THIS)**

Preventive service visits should include the age, gender appropriate history, examination, counseling, anticipatory guidance/risk factor reduction interventions, ordering lab and diagnostic screening procedures. Young children are usually seen shortly after coming home from the hospital, then at 2, 4, 6, 9, 12, 18, 24, 36, 48 and 60 months for well child visits with vaccinations. Your organization will have built into the electronic medical record (EMR) prompts for you to ask questions during these visits that capture things like normal growth and development as well as routine screenings that should be performed at each age. You will also review and provide the parent or caregiver information on anticipatory guidance, meaning information on what to expect the child to achieve by the next visit, with suggestions to enhance learning and development.

The goal of these visits is to screen for how the family is adjusting and to look at the child through a holistic lens. This includes physically assessing for any problems in growth and development, screening as recommended, and giving any immunizations which are coded separately with an educational component.

As patients progress from childhood to adulthood there are different screenings and immunizations recommended at each life stage. It is important for you as a NP to become familiar with the recommended guidelines from reliable sources such as the United Service Preventive Task Force (USPTF) https://www.uspreventiveservice staskforce.org/uspstf/ or the Centers for Disease Control (CDC) https://www.cdc.gov /vaccines/index.html to help guide you in recommending the required screenings at each age. Review the following template for a wellness visit with the various categories and example descriptions.

Table 3-4 Template of a wellness visit

Component of Documentation Well Visit	Categories	Descriptive Examples
Health history	Medical	History of hypertension
	Surgical	Cholecystectomy
	Social history	Tobacco and alcohol and illicit drug use
	Family history	Family history of cardiac disease, diabetes, cancers, chronic musculoskeletal disorders, and sudden death
Review of systems Subjective data per patient report	General	Fevers, unexpected weight changes
	Head, ears, eyes, nose, throat (HEENT)	Changes of the shape of head and scalp hair pattern; vision changes; loss of hearing; difficulty swallowing; changes in lymph nodes
	Dermatologic	Presence of any scars, rashes, or lesions
	Respiratory	Difficulty breathing, coughing, or wheezing
	Cardiovascular	Chest pain, palpitations
	Gastrointestinal	Abdominal pain, changes in bowel habits
	Endocrine	Frequent urination or increased thirst
	Hematological-immunologic	Seasonal allergies, bruising, or bleeding
	Musculoskeletal	Joint pain, stiffness or decreased range of motion
	Neurological	Numbness or tingling, headaches, seizures
	Psychiatric	Changes in mood such as depression, anxiety, behavior, memory

Physical assessment Objective findings from your physical exam	Vital signs	Temperature, pulse, respirations, blood pressure, pain scale, oxygen saturation
	General appearance	Not ill-appearing, no acute distress, dressed appropriately
	HEENT	Inspect evidence of trauma to the head, pupillary reaction, EOMs, visual acuity, presence of glasses or contacts
	Cardiovascular	Auscultation of heart sounds, PMI, peripheral pulses, lower extremity edema
	Respiratory	Inspect chest and A/P diameter, use of accessory muscles, auscultation of lung sounds
		Presence of scars, abdominal pain with palpation, auscultation of bowel sounds, percussion of liver and spleen
	Abdomen	Inspect genital skin for lesions, an inspection of penis, scrotum testicles and vagina. Rectal and anus exam
	Genitourinary	Inspect breasts for deformities, palpate lymph nodes and breast tissue for abnormalities
	Breasts	Inspect joints for stability and range of motion.
	Musculoskeletal	Assess CN II-XII; assess sensation of fingers and toes; assess
	Neurological	the strength of upper and lower extremities; assess balance and gait

(Continued)

Table 3-4 (Continued)

Component of Documentation Well Visit	Categories	Descriptive Examples
Health promotion counseling	Recommendations by US Preventative Health Services Task Force (USPSTF);	Review age-appropriate recommendations for health screening
	Immunizations per Advisory Committee on Immunization Practices (ACIP) or Centers for Disease Control (CDC)	Review immunization schedule
	Anticipatory guidance	Firearm safety; dental care; eye care; seat belt use; nutrition and weight counseling, oral care, growth and development, end of life planning

Table 3.5 New patient E/M coding

99381	*Initial comprehensive preventive medicine <1 year*
99382	*Early childhood (1–4 years)*
99383	*Late childhood (5–11 years)*
99384	*Adolescent (12–17 years)*
99385	*18–39 years*
99386	*40–64 years*
99387	*65 years or older* **(MEDICARE DOES NOT COVER THIS)**

Table 3.6 Established patient E/M coding

99391	*Initial comprehensive preventive medicine <1 year*
99392	*Early childhood (1–4 years)*
99393	*Late childhood (5–11 years)*
99394	*Adolescent (12–17 years)*
99395	*18–39 years*
99396	*40–64 years*
99397	*65 years or older* **(MEDICARE DOES NOT COVER THIS)**

EXAMPLE WELLNESS NOTE

CC: Annual Wellness exam

HPI: 42 yo female comes in for her annual wellness exam. She reports no previous problems this year and feels in good health. She had history of HTN but has lost 60 pounds and is no longer on BP medication

Past Medical History: HTN
Social History: Denies smoking, drinking or illicit drug use

ROS: General – reports loss of 60 pounds intentional weight loss
HEENT – denies visual changes
Respiratory – denies shortness of breath
Cardiac – denies palpitations, or dyspnea on exertion
Skin – denies any rashes or new moles
Muscular Skeletal – denies joint pain or back pain
Psych – denies depression or anxiety

VS: 120/80 P 80 R 16 T 98.6 Ht 5'5" Weight 135 pounds

PE: General – well developed female in no apparent distress
Respiratory – nonlabored, CTA in both lung fields
Cardiac – RRR with no murmurs or rubs
Breasts – round, symmetrical with no masses or lumps felt
GYN – normal rugae, cervix pink with no lesions or tenderness, no
drainage or odor seen, ovaries are nonpalpable

A/P

Cervical Cancer Screening – Pap test obtained.
Breast Cancer Screening – screening mammography ordered

Anticipatory guidance/counseling – discussed perimenopausal symptoms, need for increased weight bearing exercise to improve bone health and Calcium/ Vitamin D supplementation. Discussed stress reduction and good sleep hygiene.

DOCUMENTATION OF A CHRONIC DISEASE

Documentation of a chronic disease is aimed at gathering necessary information the management of different chronic diseases as follows:

Table 3.7 Chronic disease management visit

Chief complaint (CC)	What brought you here today?	Short (in patient's own words) eg. "I have a headache"
History of present illness (HPI)	Chronological order of events **INCLUDE SYSTEMIC SYMPTOMS, IS CONDITION IMPROVING, WORSENING, OR UNCHANGED? Chronic illnesses that may be affecting conditions such as COPD**	
Past medical history	Include if it is at treatment goal or not:	Example HTN is at goal of treatment BP < 140/90
Family hx	That is pertinent to CC	
Social hx	That is pertinent or needs to be considered eg. occupational hazard, daycare, smoking, drinking, recreational or illicit drug use	
Allergies		
Medications	Include herbs and over the counter medications	
Review of systems (ROS)	General	Any fevers, gained or lost weight
Subjective data	Hair, skin, & nails	Is hair dry or oily, skin changes
You ask questions to uncover more detail patient confirms or denies	Head	
	Neck	Any lymph nodes enlarged

(Continued)

Table 3.7 (Continud)

	Eyes	Any visual changes
	Ears	Any hearing changes, pain in ear
	Nose	Any drainage
	Mouth & throat	Do they have a sore throat. Any lesions in their mouth
	Cardiovascular	Any chest pain or palpitations
	Respiratory	Any shortness of breath, wheezing
	Breasts	Any lumps or masses in breasts
	Gastrointestinal	Any nausea/vomiting/diarrhea
	Musculoskeletal	Any joint pain
	Peripheral	Any swelling
	Neurological	Any numbness, tingling, dizziness
	Psychiatric	Any mood changes

Vital signs (VS)	BP P R T pulse oximetry Height Weight BMI	
Physical exam (PE) – Objective data you examine or observe	General	How do they look overall?
	Hair, skin, & nails	Any skin lesions noted, nails blunted?
	Head	Symmetrical
	Neck	Any lymph nodes enlarged?
	Eyes	Sclera/conjunctiva
	Ears	What does tympanic membrane look like?
	Nose	Any drainage?
	Mouth & throat	Any lesions? Look at tonsils
	Cardiovascular	Rate and rhythm of heart/any murmurs
	Respiratory	What do their lungs sound like?
	Breasts	Any lumps or masses felt?
	Gastrointestinal	Any abdominal tenderness, bowel sounds?
	Musculoskeletal	Can they move all their joints, any swelling?
	Peripheral	Any pedal edema? How is circulation?
	Neurological	How is their gait, sensation, balance?
	Psychiatric	Are they appropriate with good insight?
Labs reviewed	Include creatine clearance if known for medication dosing	

(Continued)

Table 3.7 (Continud)

Radiology reviewed		
Independent interpretations	*Include if you independently interpreted the results (EKG, CXR), do not include if it will be billed somewhere else*	
Chronic disease(s)	*List in rank order/list plan such as future tests, medications*	1 2 3
Education/follow up	**What will you educate the patient about and when should they follow up?**	
External records reviewed	*Did you review records outside of your practice for this encounter? Labs/tests/other provider notes?*	
Independent historian	*Did you obtain information regarding history from someone other than the patient due to mental status, age, or condition to help you in MDM?*	

Collaboration	Discussion of management with external clinicians or appropriate source	
Shared decision making	Testing or treatment considered, even if not done	
Social determinants of health	Conditions that may influence patients' conditions (inability to fill prescriptions, transportation, insufficient insurance)	
Decision to hospitalize	If considered give reason why or why not	
Code status	Decision to de-escalate care because of poor prognosis patient/family wishes	

EXAMPLE OF CHRONIC OFFICE VISIT NOTE

CC: "My blood sugars have been running low"

HPI: 68 yo male lives alone, h/o dementia x 3 years which appears to be worsening per daughter and type 2 diabetes x 10 years, last hemoglobin A1c in hospital 3 months ago was 7.5. Pt was hospitalized at that time for cellulitis which has since cleared. Now with complaints of feeling dizzy and faint at times which is relieved with food. Noted change in Levemir dosage from last hospital visit from 15 units at HS to 20 units. Daughter reports she is unclear if patient is dosing medication at night correctly because blood sugars have been very inconsistent.

PMH: Dementia
Sox hx: Smokes 1 ppd for 40 years
Allergies: NKA
Medications:
   Metformin 500mg twice a day
   Levemir 20 units at night
ROS:
   General – no reports of weight gained or lost
   Cardiac – no c/o chest pain
   Respiratory – no c/o shortness of breath
   GI – no c/o diarrhea or changes in stool
   GU – reports increased urination but no burning
   Neuro – c/o feeling light-headed like he is going to pass out
PE:
   VS – 120/80 P 80 R16
   General – elderly gentleman who appears unkept
   Cardiac – normal rate and rhythm with no murmurs
   GI – soft nontender with normal bowel sounds
   Neurological – decreased sensation on both feet
   Skin – no lesions noted
   Psy – alert x 3 and appropriate with diminished insight

A/P
1. Diabetes
    Reviewed home blood sugar logs
    Reviewed last hemoglobin A1c at hospital
    Ordered hemoglobin A1c
    Adjusted dosage of insulin to Levemir 15 units at HS
2. Dementia – Slums test given in office with moderate signs of dementia present

Education: Discussed allowing a higher hemoglobin A1c per American Diabetic Guidelines due to age and comorbidities with a target of HbA1c of < 8.5
    Total time spent in encounter, including review of outside records, face-to-face time, ordering tests, prescriptions, and completion of documentation 45 minutes.

DOCUMENTATION OF AN ACUTE DISEASE

Documentation of an acute disease is aimed at gathering the necessary information to be able to determine what the differential diagnoses are and come up with a plan.

EXAMPLE OF ACUTE OFFICE VISIT NOTE

CC: "My throat hurts and my body aches. I have chills and probably a fever."
    HPI: Patient complaint of sore throat x 3 days. Sore throat pain is 8/10 on pain scale and has interfered with drinking and eating. Patient states swallowing liquids or solids aggravates pain. Patient using throat lozenges to alleviate pain which lessens pain to 6/10 on pain scale for short periods of time. Patient states body aches started 3 days ago that accompanied her sore throat. States she feels "weak" which has interfered with her daily activities. She states body aches

are generalized and cannot pinpoint exact area of aching. Patient states she has had chills for 2 days. Client has been febrile.

PMH: Occasional colds

Sox hx: Works full time at the Boys and Girls Club as an activity coordinator

Allergies: NKA

Medications:

Albuterol HFA 108mcg albuterol sulfate 2 puffs every 4 hours as needed

ROS:

GENERAL: Complaints of body aches and fatigue for 3 days. Fever and chills "off and on" for 2 days. Highest temperature 102.1F last pm at 2000

NOSE: Denies congestion, discharge

THROAT/MOUTH: Complains of sore throat and complains of throat feeling "swollen". States throat pain is an 8/10 on pain scale and is worse when she tries to eat or drink. Patient states her throat pain is also causing neck pain. States pain in throat for 3 days "getting worse every day".

NECK: States her neck glands are swollen and painful to the touch. Denies goiter, neck stiffness or pain upon movement of neck.

RESP: Non-productive cough for the last 1–2 days. Complains of SOB with moderate exertion. Denies need for albuterol inhaler use. Denies dyspnea.

PE:

GENERAL: Well-groomed, 30-year-old female, who does not look like she feels well

HEAD: Frontal and maxillary sinuses without pain on palpation

EARS: Tympanic membrane pearly gray with no bulging, redness, or distortion bilat.

NOSE: Nares are patent bilaterally with no noted congestion

THROAT/MOUTH: Tonsils are intact. Edema and erythema are noted. Gray exudate is noted on tonsils bilaterally. Grade 3+ swelling is noted. Posterior pharynx pink and moist with a small amount of patchy, gray exudate. Uvula with mild erythema, without deviation
NECK: Tonsillar and anterior cervical lymphadenopathy and tenderness noted
RESP: Lungs clear to auscultation bilaterally. Respiratory excursion is symmetrical

Tests:
Used the guideline "Clinical Decision Rule for Management of Sore Throat" (AAFP, 2009)
Scored as follows:

- Absence of cough=1
- Swollen and tender anterior cervical lymph nodes=1
- Temperature >100.4=0
- Tonsillar exudate or swelling=1
- Age 15–44=0

Score=3 Throat culture/RADT
　Positive – Treat with antibiotics

Rapid antigen test for group A Streptococcus done in office and was positive, influenza neg.

Differentials considered – strep pharyngitis, viral pharyngitis, influenza, sinusitis, mononucleosis.

A/P
　Strep pharyngitis
- Amoxicillin 875mg orally Bid for 10 days
- Acetaminophen 650 mg orally every 4 to 6 hours as needed for pain or fever. Do not exceed 4g in a 24-hour period

- - Ibuprofen 600mg orally every 6 hours as needed for pain or fever
  - Education
- Medication side effects
  - Amoxicillin-nausea, vomiting, diarrhea, urticaria, rash, black hairy tongue, yeast infection
  - Ibuprofen-nausea, headache, rash, tinnitus, GI upset
  - Tylenol-nausea, rash, headache
- Supportive care
  - Rest
  - Fluids
  - Cold drinks and popsicles
  - Throat lozenges as needed
- Complete the full antibiotic course even if she is feeling better
- Symptoms will usually resolve within 3–4 days
- Eat yogurt at least once daily to counter some of the side effects of the antibiotic
- Take antibiotic and ibuprofen with food or milk to lessen GI symptoms
- No work or school until 24 hours after the first dose of antibiotics because strep is infectious until 24 hours after the antibiotic is first started
- No kissing or sharing utensils
- Change toothbrush to prevent reinfection
- Good hand washing technique and proper cough/cover instruction
- Follow up for this condition as needed. For worsening symptoms or adverse reactions to medications, return to PCP, urgent care, or ER for treatment
- Follow up with PCP regarding 2nd MMR and tetanus booster

As you can see from the above documentation, the history of present illness, ROS, and PE were much more extensive than what was required for coding and billing purposes. A medically appropriate history and physical exam are whatever the clinician decides is necessary in order for them to decide on the diagnosis and the plan of care.

Table 3.8 Template for documenting an acute disease

Chief complaint (CC)	What brought you here today?	Short (in patient's own words) eg. "I have a headache"
History of present illness (HPI)	Chronological order of events, before onset of CC, must include OLDCARTS in paragraph form **INCLUDE SYSTEMIC SYMPTOMS, IS CONDITION IMPROVING, WORSENING, OR UNCHANGED; Chronic illnesses that may be affecting conditions such as COPD**	
	Onset	
	Location	
	Duration	
	Character	
	Aggravating/associated factors	
	Relieving factors	
	Temporal factors – other things going on	
	Severity	
Past medical history	Include if it is at treatment goal or not: Example HTN is at goal of treatment BP < 140/90	
Family hx	Pertinent to CC	
Social hx	Pertinent or needs to be considered eg. In MDM. Examples: Occupational hazard, daycare, smoking, drinking, recreational or illicit drug use	

(Continued)

Table 3.8 (Continued)

Allergies		
Medications	Include herbs and over the counter medications	
Review of systems (ROS)	General	*Any fevers, gained or lost weight?*
	Hair, skin, & nails	*Is hair dry or oily, skin changes?*
Subjective data	Head	
You ask questions to uncover more detail.	Neck	*Any lymph nodes enlarged?*
Patient confirms or denies symptoms	Eyes	*Any visual changes?*
	Ears	*Any hearing changes, pain in ear?*
	Nose	*Any drainage?*
	Mouth & throat	*Do they have a sore throat? Any lesions in their mouth?*
	Cardiovascular	*Any chest pain or palpitations?*
	Respiratory	*Any shortness of breath, wheezing?*
	Breasts	*Any lumps or masses in breasts?*
	Gastrointestinal	*Any nausea/vomiting/diarrhea?*
	Musculoskeletal	*Any joint pain?*
	Peripheral	*Any swelling?*
	Neurological	*Any numbness, tingling, dizziness?*
	Psychiatric	*Any mood changes?*

Vital signs (VS)	BP P R T pulse oximetry Height Weight BMI	
Physical exam(PE) – Objective data you examine or observe	General	How do they look overall!?
	Hair, skin, & nails	Any skin lesions noted, nails blunted?
	Head	Symmetrical
	Neck	Any lymph nodes enlarged?
	Eyes	Sclera/Conjunctiva
	Ears	What does tympanic membrane look like?
	Nose	Any drainage?
	Mouth & throat	Any lesions? Look at tonsils
	Cardiovascular	Rate and rhythm of heart/any murmurs?
	Respiratory	What do their lungs sound like?
	Breasts	Any lumps or masses felt?
	Gastrointestinal	Any abdominal tenderness, bowel sounds?
	Musculoskeletal	Can they move all their joints, any swelling?
	Peripheral	Any pedal edema? How is circulation?
	Neurological	How is their gait, sensation, balance?
	Psychiatric	Are they appropriate with good insight?

(Continued)

Table 3.8 (Continued)

Labs reviewed	Include creatine clearance if known for medication dosing
Radiology reviewed	
Independent interpretations	Include if you independently interpreted the results (EKG, CXR) unless this will be billed separately elsewhere such as by radiology
Differential diagnosis/ plan	List in rank order with symptoms that support it as well as what tests you will do to rule in/out 1 2 3
Diagnosis/plan	Rank order if more than 1 and include your plan – tests, medications etc.
Education/follow up	What will you educate patient on and when do you want them to follow up?
External records reviewed	Did you review records outside of your practice for this encounter? Labs/tests/ other provider notes?
Independent historian	Did you obtain information regarding history from someone other than the patient due to mental status, age, or condition to help you in MDM?
Collaboration	Discussion of management with external clinicians or appropriate source

Shared decision making	*Testing or treatment considered, even if not done*	
Social determinants of health	*Conditions that may influence patient's conditions (inability to fill prescriptions, transportation, insufficient insurance)*	
Decision to hospitalize	*If considered state, why or why not?*	
Code status	*Decision to de-escalate care because of poor prognosis patient/family wishes*	

DOCUMENTATION OF A MEDICARE ANNUAL WELLNESS VISIT

Once patients turn 65, providers can no longer bill for a "wellness visit" *because Medicare will not pay for these exams.* These visits may be covered under *private insurance* but by statute Medicare cannot pay for a visit that does not include managing a chronic illness, complaint, or injury. If you code for a wellness exam the patient will be liable for the bill.

Medicare does have specific preventive screening exams that are meant to be helpful at screening and preventing diseases. These visits are not the annual physical exam; they are preventive wellness exams thus they do not include management of chronic conditions, testing, or an extensive physical exam. *This visit is meant to review, screen, and plan for the following year the preventive health activities advised. Before the visit make sure the patient gathers the following documents:*

- Medical records to include immunization record
- Family history
- All medication they are taking to include supplements
- All providers they have seen that are involved in their care with contact information

The following forms can be used for documentation of each visit and include all the necessary parts.

Table 3.9 Template for recording initial preventative physical exam (IPPE)

G0402 – Initial preventive physical exam (IPPE)	New to Medicare (within first 12 months of Medicare Part B)
Review patient's medical and social history	*PMH*
	Soc hx
	Fam hx
	Medications (including supplements)
	Diet/Physical activity
	ETOH screening, tobacco, and recreational or illicit drugs

Table 3.9 (Continued)

Screening	*Depression*
Functional status	*Hearing*
	Fall risk
	Home safety
	Ability to perform ADLs
Exam	*Vital signs, BMP*
	Visual acuity screen
	Any other screening deemed appropriate
End of life planning	*Discuss end of life planning − with verbal and written component*
Review opioid prescription if appropriate	*Review for opioid use disorder risk factors*
	Evaluate pain and severity with current treatment plan
	Provide non-opioid treatment options information
	Refer to a specialist if needed
Screen for potential substance use disorder (SUD)	*Review the patient's potential for SUD and refer if needed. This tool is available per NIH but is not required*
	https://nida.nih.gov/ nidamed-medical-health-professionals/ screening-tools-resources/chart-screening-tools
Educate, counsel, and refer as needed	*Based on your assessment provide appropriate education, counseling, and referrals*
Educate, counsel, and refer for other preventive services	*A written plan like a checklist the patient can follow*
	Once in a lifetime EKG, as appropriate
	Appropriate screenings/vaccinations as recommended

Table 3.10 Template for recording initial annual wellness visit

G-0438: Initial annual wellness visit (AMV)

Health risk assessment
Medical and family history
List of current providers
Measure
Assess cognition
Screen for depression
Review functional ability
Written schedule
Primary/secondary/tertiary recommendations
Provide appropriate advice, counseling, and referrals
Provide advance care planning services
Review current opioid prescriptions
Screen for potential substance use disorders

Table 3.11 Template for recording subsequent annual wellness visits

G-0439: Subsequent annual wellness visits (AMV)

Review and update health risk assessment
Update medical and family history
Update list of current providers
Measure – weight, BP, routine measures as deemed appropriate
Assess cognition
Update patient's written screening schedule
Update primary/secondary/tertiary recommendations
Provide appropriate advice, counseling, and referrals
Provide advance care planning services
Review current opioid prescriptions
Screen for potential substance use disorders

EVALUATION AND MANAGEMENT CODING CHANGES 2021/2023

The changes in 2021 were so successful that in 2023 they replaced the 1995/1997 rules *across all places of service. In 2021 the history category and the exam category were no longer a part of the coding process which significantly simplified billing which only depended now on the medical decision-making piece, however providers still needed to document a pertinent history and exam. These changes remained in effect with the 2023 changes.* The 2023 E/M changes included 93 revisions, 75 deletions, and 225 new codes all of which took place on January 1, 2023.

Table 4.1 E/M 2021/2023 Billing structure for new office visit

E/M code	History	Exam	MDM	Time	Reimbursement
99202	*History and physical exam should be appropriate as determined by the physician and is no longer calculated into billing*		*Straightforward*	15–29	$72.86*
99203			*Low Complexity*	30–44	$112.84*
99204			*Mod Complexity*	45–59	$167.40*
99205			*High Complexity*	60–74	$220.95*

*Per the 2023 Medicare Physician Fee Schedule (Centers for Medicare and Medicaid Services [CMS], 2023)

DOI: 10.4324/9781003542872-4

Table 4.2 E/M 2021/2023 Billing structure for established office visit

E/M code	History	Exam	MDM	Time	Reimbursement
99211	History and physical exam should be appropriate as determined by the physician and is no longer calculated into billing		None	NA	$23.38*
99212			Straightforward	10–19	$56.93*
99213			Low Complexity	20–29	$90.82*
99214			Mod Complexity	30–39	$128.43*
99215			High Complexity	40–54	$179.94*

*Per the 2023 Medicare Physician Fee Schedule (CMS, 2023)

Notice the 99211 level of service does not require any medical decision making or time requirement. Per the CPT guidelines the 99211-billing code is for "Outpatient visits of an established patient, that may not require the presence of a physician. Usually, the presenting problem(s) are minimal" (AAPC Thought Leadership Team, 2024).

99211 REQUIREMENTS

- Must be a face-to-face interaction
- Must have an E/M service performed
- Physician does not need to be present
- It must be an established patient

The 99211 level of service is ***mainly*** for nurses' visits. Examples include BP checks, TB skin tests, simple dressing changes, urinalysis for a urinary tract infection, PT/INR for coumadin dose adjustment, calibrating a glucose meter or supervised drug screen, removing sutures, etc. To claim a 99211, the person who performed the service must document the E/M service in the medical record. Here is an example of a note for a 99211 documented by the registered nurse.

Table 4.3 NEW E/M 2023 medical decision-making tool

MDM (Based on 2 out of 3 elements of MDM)	COPA	DATA	RISK
99211	N/A	N/A	N/A
Straightforward 99202 99212 99221 99231 99234	1 self-limited or minor problem	Minimal or NONE	Minimal risk of morbidity from additional diagnostic testing or treatment
Low complexity 99203 99213 99221 99231 99234	2 or more self-limited or minor problems, or 1 stable, chronic illness, or 1 acute uncomplicated illness or injury or 1 stable, acute illness	(Must meet 1 of 2 requirements) **Category 1: Tests and documents** Any combination of 2 from the following • Review of prior external note(s) from each unique source • Review of the result(s) of each unique test • Ordering of each unique test	Low risk of morbidity from additional diagnostic testing or treatment

(Continued)

Table 4.3 (Continued)

MDM

(Based on 2 out of 3 elements of MDM)	COPA	DATA	RISK
	or *1 acute, uncomplicated illness or injury requiring hospital inpatient or observation level of care*	**or** **Category 2: Assessment requiring an independent historian(s)**	
Moderate 99204 99214 99222 99232 99235	*1 or more chronic illnesses with exacerbation, progression, or side effects of treatment* **or** *2 or more stable chronic illnesses* **or** *1 undiagnosed new problem with uncertain prognosis*	*(Must meet 1 out of 3 requirements)* **Category 1: Tests, documents, historian** *Any combination of 3 from the following* • *Review of prior external note(s) from each unique source* • *Review of the result(s) of each unique test* • *Ordering of each unique test* • *Assessment requiring an independent historian(s)*	*Moderate risk of morbidity from additional diagnostic testing or treatment* Examples only: • *Prescription drug management* • *Decision regarding minor surgery with identified patient or procedure risk factors*

	or *1 acute illness with systemic symptoms* *or* *1 acute, complicated injury*	*or* **Category 2: Independent interpretation of tests** • *Independent interpretation of a test performed by another physician/other qualified healthcare professional (not separately reported)* *or* **Category 3: Discussion of management or test interpretation.** • *Discussion of management or test interpretation with external/physician/ other qualified healthcare professional/ appropriate source (not separately reported)*	• *Decision regarding elective major surgery without identified patient or procedure risk factors.* • *Diagnosis or treatment significantly limited by social determinants of health*
High complexity 99205 99215 99223 99233 99236	*1 or more chronic illnesses with severe exacerbation, progression, or side effects of treatment* *or* *1 acute or chronic illness or injury that poses a threat to life or bodily function*	*(Must meet 2 out of 3 requirements)* **Category 1: Tests, documents, historian** *Any combination of 3 from the following* • *Review of prior external note(s) from each unique source* • *Review of the result(s) of each unique test* • *Ordering of each unique test* • *Assessment requiring an independent historian(s)*	*High risk of morbidity from additional diagnostic testing or treatment* *Examples only:* • *Drug therapy requiring intensive monitoring for toxicity.*

(Continued)

Table 4.3 (Continued)

MDM (Based on 2 out of 3 elements of MDM)	COPA	DATA	RISK
	or *Multiple morbidities requiring intensive management (initial nursing facility only)*	**or** **Category 2: Independent interpretation of tests** • *Independent interpretation of a test performed by another physician/other qualified healthcare professional (not separately reported)* **or** **Category 3: Discussion of management or test interpretation** • *Discussion of management or test interpretation with external/physician/other qualified healthcare professional/appropriate source (not separately reported)*	• *Decision for elective major surgery with identified patient or procedure risk factors* • *Decision for emergency major surgery* • *Decision regarding hospitalization* • *Decision for DNR or to de-escalate care because of poor prognosis* • *Parenteral controlled substances*

Source: American Medical Association, 2022

Table 4.4 Example of a 99211 nurse visit:

CC	*"I need my BP rechecked"*
HPI	*36-year-old male here for BP recheck after recently being started on BP medication 2 weeks ago*
PFSH	
ROS	*No c/o headache or dizziness*
PE	*BP 104/80*
A/P	*Performed by Jane Doe, RN, message sent to provider*

The 2023 revisions include codes for the following places of service (99202–99499)

- Office New and Established or other outpatient services (99202–99215)
- Hospital Inpatient and Observation (99221–99239)
- Emergency Department Services (99281–99285)
- Nursing Facility Services (99304–99316)
- Home or Residence Services (99341–99350)

(American Medical Association, 2022)

Now, let's look at the new 2023 MDM tool one element at a time starting with the number and complexity of problems addressed at the encounter (COPA).

Table 4.5 #1 COPA: Number and complexity of problems addressed

Level of MDM Based on 2 out of 3	Number and complexity of problems addressed at the encounter (COPA)	Amount and complexity of data to be reviewed or analyzed (DATA)	Risk of complications and/or morbidity or mortality of patient management (RISK)

COPA DEFINITIONS

- Problem – defined as the reason you came to the clinic or facility
- Managing a problem – involves actively managing or considering options for a particular problem that is documented
- Chronic problem – a problem that is expected to last at least one year or until the patient dies
- Stable problem – a problem where the treatment goal has been reached. For example, you have DM type 2 and your hemoglobin A1c is 6. Your goal hemoglobin A1c is 6.5. Your diabetes is considered stable. **TIP:** Be sure to document what the goal for each condition is so you can determine if the problem is stable or unstable
- Unstable problem – a problem where the treatment goal has NOT been reached. For example, you have HTN, and your goal BP is < 140/90 but your BP today is 160/85. Your goal BP has not been reached so this problem would be considered unstable
- Comorbidities – chronic conditions are NOT considered UNLESS they are affecting the current problem AND are addressed in the note
- Differentials should be listed as they are KEY elements in determining COPA

Source: American Medical Association, 2022

Table 4.6 #1 COPA – Problems addressed

MDM	COPA
99211	N/A
Straightforward (SF)	1 self-limited or minor problem
Low	2 or more self-limited or minor problems,
	or
	1 stable, chronic illness,
	or
	1 acute uncomplicated illness or injury
	or
	1 stable, acute illness
	or
	1 acute, uncomplicated illness or injury requiring hospital inpatient or observation level of care

Table 4.6 #1 (Continued)

Moderate	1 or more chronic illnesses with exacerbation, progression, or side effects of treatment,
	or
	2 or more stable chronic illnesses
	or
	1 undiagnosed new problem with uncertain prognosis
	or
	1 acute illness with systemic symptoms
	or
	1 acute, complicated injury
High	1 or more chronic illnesses with severe exacerbation, progression, or side effects of treatment
	or
	1 acute or chronic illness or injury that poses a threat to life or bodily function
	or
	Multiple morbidities requiring intensive management (initial nursing facility only)

Source: American Medical Association, 2022

Table 4.7 Example: Straightforward (COPA)

MDM	Number and complexity of problems Addressed at the encounter (COPA)	Definition
SF	1 self-limited or minor problem	A problem that will run a definite and prescribed course that is transient in nature such as the common cold

Table 4.8 Example: Low Complexity (COPA)

MDM	Number and Complexity Of Problems Addressed at the encounter (COPA)	Definition
Low	2 or more self-limited or minor problems	Two or more problems that run a definite and prescribed course that are transient in nature and not likely to permanently alter the health status of the individual
	1 stable, chronic illness	A stable chronic illness is one in which the treatment goal has been reached
	1 acute uncomplicated illness or injury	This is a recent short-term problem which carries a low risk of morbidity for which you are considering treatment. There is little risk of mortality with treatment, and you expect a full recovery with no impairment
	1 stable, acute illness (resolution may not be complete)	This is a new or recent problem such as pneumonia and you have started the patient on treatment and they are improving, but treatment and resolution may not be complete; it is considered stable at this time
	1 acute, uncomplicated illness or injury requiring hospital inpatient or observation level of care	This is a new short-term problem that carries a low risk of morbidity for which treatment is required. There is little or no risk of mortality with treatment and you expect full recovery without functional impairment. However, the treatment required is delivered in a hospital inpatient or observation level setting

Source: American Medical Association, 2022

Table 4.9 Example: Moderate (COPA)

MDM	Number and complexity of problems Addressed at the encounter (COPA)	Definition
Moderate	1 or more chronic illnesses with exacerbation, progression, or side effects of treatment	*This is a chronic illness such as COPD that is acutely worsening, poorly controlled or progressing with the intent to improve the overall condition through supportive care or requiring attention due to side effects*
	2 or more stable chronic illnesses	*This is the patient who has two or more conditions that you are managing that are at goal*
	1 undiagnosed new problem with uncertain prognosis	*This is a problem that is in the* **DIFFERENTIAL** *list that represents something that could result in morbidity if left untreated. Examples include MI for chest pain, PE for SOB, DVT for leg swelling etc.*
	1 acute illness with systemic symptoms	*This is an illness that causes systemic symptoms and has a high risk of morbidity without treatment such as hypoxia, low blood pressure, or sepsis. Symptoms such as fever, body aches, or fatigue in a minor illness that could be treated should not count.*
	1 acute, complicated injury	*This is an injury that requires treatment that includes evaluation of body systems that are not directly part of the injured organ, the injury is extensive, or the treatment options are multiple and associated with risk of morbidity. This could include a head injury or complicated fracture, car accident etc.*

Source: American Medical Association, 2022

Table 4.10 Example: High

MDM	Number and complexity of problems addressed at the encounter (COPA)	Definitions
High	1 or more chronic illnesses with severe exacerbation, progression, or side effects of treatment	Severe exacerbation or progression of a chronic illness or severe side effects of treatment that have a significant risk of morbidity and may require escalation in level of care.
	1 acute or chronic illness or injury that poses a threat to life or bodily function	An acute illness with systemic symptoms, or an acute complicated injury or a chronic illness or injury with exacerbation and or progression or side effects of treatment that pose a threat to life or bodily function in the near term without treatment. Some symptoms may represent a condition that is significantly probable and poses a potential threat to life or bodily function.
	Multiple morbidities requiring intensive management (initial nursing facility only)	This is a set of conditions, syndromes or functional impairments that are likely to require frequent medication changes or other treatment changes and/or re-evaluations. The patient is at significant risk of worsening medical status, (including behavioral) and risk for (re)admission to a hospital.

Source: American Medical Association, 2022

Table 4.11 #2 DATA reviewed or analyzed

LEVEL of MDM Based on 2 out of 3	Number and complexity of problems addressed at the encounter **(COPA)**	Amount and complexity of data to be reviewed or analyzed **(DATA)**	Risk of complications and/or morbidity or mortality of patient management **(RISK)**

DATA DEFINITIONS

- Analysis – the process of using the data as part of the medical decision-making process, for example, analyzing the hemoglobin trend in acute blood loss anemia to guide decisions for blood transfusion.
- Test – includes imaging, laboratory, psychometric, or physiologic data (pulse oximetry is NOT considered a test).
- Unique test – defined by the CPT code set. If multiple results of the same unique test are analyzed, for example serial hemoglobins they count as one test, also if you have overlapping tests they only count as one, for example a CBC and an H/H are overlapping.
- Unique Source – a clinician outside of your practice.
- External records –records, communications, and or tests that come from an external source outside of your practice. Reviewing notes previously from your practice does not count.
- Discussion – requires an interactive exchange. This exchange must be direct and have occurred within a day or two. Sending chart notes or written exchanges that are within progress notes does not qualify as an interactive exchange. The discussion must reflect that it is part of the MDM process for the patient.
- Independent historian – an individual such as a parent, guardian, surrogate, spouse, or witness that provides additional information to the history provided by the patient who is unable to provide a complete or reliable history. This does NOT include translator services.

- Independent interpretation – the interpretation of a test for which there is a CPT code, and a report is customary. This interpretation should be documented but does not need to be a formal or complete report of the test. It should also not be billed separately when it is a test the radiologist will interpret and bill for.
- Appropriate source – an appropriate source includes professionals who are not in the healthcare profession but may be involved in the management of the patient such as a social worker, case manager, parole officer, lawyer, teacher etc. It does not include family or informed caregivers.

(American Medical Association, 2022)

Table 4.12 #2 Amount and complexity of data to be reviewed (DATA)

MDM (Based on 2 out of 3 elements of MDM)	Complexity of data reviewed
99211	*N/A*
Straightforward	*Minimal or none*
LOW complexity	*(Must meet 1 of 2 requirements)*
	Category 1: Tests and documents
	Any combination of 2 from the following
	• *Review of prior external note(s) from each unique source*
	• *Review of the result(s) of each unique test*
	• *Ordering of each unique test*
	OR
	Category 2: Assessment requiring an independent historian(s)

Table 4.12 (Continued)

Moderate	*(Must meet 1 out of 3 requirements)* **Category 1: Tests, documents, historian** *Any combination of 3 from the following* • *Review of prior external note(s) from each unique source* • *Review of the result(s) of each unique test* • *Ordering of each unique test* • *Assessment requiring an independent historian(s)* **or** **Category 2: Independent interpretation of tests** • *Independent interpretation of a test performed by another physician/other qualified healthcare professional not separately reported.* **or** **Category 3: Discuss of management or test interpretation** • *Discussion of management or test interpretation with external/physician/other qualified healthcare professional/appropriate source (not separately reported)*
High complexity	*(Must meet 2 out of 3 requirements)* **Category 1: Tests, documents, historian** *Any combination of 3 from the following* • *Review of prior external note(s) from each unique source* • *Review of the result(s) of each unique test* • *Ordering of each unique test* • *Assessment requiring an independent historian(s)* **or** **Category 2: Independent interpretation of tests** • *Independent interpretation of a test performed by another physician/other qualified healthcare professional not separately reported* **or** **Category 3: Discussion of management or test interpretation** • *Discussion of management or test interpretation with external/physician/other qualified healthcare professional/appropriate source (not separately reported)*

Table 4-13 Example: Low complexity – DATA

MDM	Complexity of data reviewed	Definitions
Low	(Must meet 1 of 2 requirements) **Category 1: Tests and documents** *Any combination of 2 from the following* • *Review of prior external note(s) from each unique source* • *Review of the result(s) of each unique test* • *Ordering of each unique test* **Category 2: Assessment requiring an independent historian(s)**	• *External notes come from outside your practice.* • *Unique source is a clinician outside of your practice.* • *Review EACH unique test – (imaging, laboratory, psychometric, or physiologic data).* • *Ordering of tests includes reviewing that result – this may include tests considered to be ordered but after shared decision making are not ordered – for example the PSA.* *Alternately you may consider a test that is normally ordered for a patient but decide against it because of the risk to the patient.* *THESE CONSIDERATIONS MUST BE DOCUMENTED TO BE COUNTED* *An independent historian is a parent, guardian, surrogate, spouse, or witness who provides additional history when patient is unable to due to developmental stage, dementia, psychosis, intubation etc.* *IT DOES NOT INCLUDE TRANSLATION SERVICES*

Table 4.14 Example: Medium complexity – DATA

MDM	Complexity of data reviewed	Definitions
Medium	**(Must meet 1 out of 3 requirements)** **Category 1: Tests, documents, historian** *Any combination of 3 from the following* • *Review of prior external note(s) from each* **unique source** • *Review of the result(s) of each* **unique test** • *Ordering of each* **unique test** • **Assessment requiring an independent historian(s)**	• *External notes come from outside your practice.* • *Unique source is a clinician outside of your practice.* • *Review EACH unique test – (imaging, laboratory, psychometric, or physiologic data).* • *Ordering of tests includes reviewing that result – this may include tests considered to be ordered but after shared decision making are not ordered – for example the PSA.* • *Alternately you may consider a test that is normally ordered for a patient but decide against it because of the risk to the patient.* • *An independent historian is a parent, guardian, surrogate, spouse, or witness who provides additional history when patient is unable to due to developmental stage, dementia, psychosis, intubation etc.* *IT DOES NOT INCLUDE TRANSLATION SERVICES*

(Continued)

Table 4-14 (Continued)

MDM	Complexity of data reviewed	Definitions
	Category 2: Independent interpretation of tests • Independent interpretation of a test performed by another physician/other qualified health care professional (not separately reported)	*The interpretation of a test for which there is a CPT code, and an interpretation or report is customary such as with an EKG or CXR. You must document your interpretation during the encounter. This should not be counted if the professional interpretation is coded separately.*
	Category 3: Discussion of management or test interpretation • Discussion of management or test interpretation with external physician/other qualified healthcare professional/appropriate source (not separately reported)	*An external clinician is an individual who is not in the same group practice or is of a different specialty or subspecialty. It is not a professional that is practicing independently. For example, if an ER physician is calling to admit a patient to your group that would count, or if you were talking to a cardiologist and discussing the echocardiogram results that would count.*

Table 4.15 Example – High complexity DATA

MDM	Complexity of data reviewed	Definitions
High	**(Must meet 2 out of 3 requirements) Category 1: Tests, documents, historian** *Any combination of 3 from the following* • *Review of prior external note(s) from each unique source* • *Review of the result(s) of each unique test* • *Ordering of each unique test* • *Assessment requiring an independent historian(s)*	• *External notes come from outside your practice.* • *Unique source is a clinician outside of your practice.* • *Review EACH unique test – (imaging, laboratory, psychometric, or physiologic data).* • *Ordering of tests includes reviewing that result – this may include tests considered to be ordered but after shared decision making are not ordered – for example the PSA.* • *Alternately you may consider a test that is normally ordered for a patient but decide against it because of the risk to the patient.* • *An independent historian is a parent, guardian, surrogate, spouse, or witness who provides additional history when patient is unable to due to developmental stage, dementia, psychosis, intubation etc.* *IT DOES NOT INCLUDE TRANSLATION SERVICES*

(Continued)

Table 4-15 (Continued)

MDM	Complexity of data reviewed	Definitions
	Category 2: Independent interpretation of tests • Independent interpretation of a test performed by another physician/other qualified healthcare professional not separately reported)	*The interpretation is of a test for which there is a CPT code, and an interpretation or report is customary such as with an EKG or CXR. You must document your interpretation during the encounter. This should not be counted if the professional interpretation is coded separately.*
	Category 3: Discussion of management or test interpretation • Discussion of management or test interpretation with external/physician/ other qualified healthcare professional/appropriate source (not separately reported)	*An external clinician is an individual who is not in the same group practice or is of a different specialty or subspecialty. It is not a professional that is practicing independently. For example, if an ER physician is calling to admit a patient to your group that would count, or if you were talking to a cardiologist and discussing the echocardiogram results that would count.*

Table 4.16 #3 RISK category

Level of MDM Based on 2 out of 3	Number and complexity of problems addressed at the encounter (COPA)	Amount and complexity of data to be reviewed or analyzed (DATA)	Risk of complications and/ or morbidity or mortality of patient management (RISK)

RISK DEFINITIONS (AMERICAN MEDICAL ASSOCIATION, 2022)

- Assessment of level of risk – this is affected by the nature of the event.
- Level of risk – this is based upon the consequences of the problems you are addressing when treated appropriately.
- Risk of patient management criteria – applies to patient management decisions made by the reporting clinician as part of the reported encounter.
- Risk also includes the medical decision making needed to initiate or forego further testing, treatment, and/or hospitalization.

Shared decision making involves eliciting the patient and/or family preferences. Provide patient and/or family education and explain the risk and benefits of the management options. Examples might include an older patient who has atrial fibrillation who should be on an oral anticoagulant to prevent strokes but is falling frequently. In this case you would discuss the benefits and risks with the patient and/or family and come to a decision based on those considerations. The decision may be to continue or stop the oral anticoagulant. Either decision is fine and would still count as shared decision making if it is documented.

Table 4.17 #3 Risk of complications and/or morbidity or mortality of patient management

MDM (Based on 2 out of 3 elements of MDM)	Risk of complications and or morbidity
99211	N/A
Straightforward	*Minimal risk of morbidity from additional diagnostic testing or treatment* **Examples only** • *Rest* • *Gargles* • *Elastic bandages* • *Superficial dressings*
Low complexity	*Low risk of morbidity from additional diagnostic testing or treatment* **Examples only** • *Over the counter (OTC) drugs* • *Minor surgery with no identified patient or procedure risk factors* • *Physical therapy* • *Occupational therapy* • *IV fluids without additives*

Moderate   *Moderate risk of morbidity from additional diagnostic testing or treatment*

Examples only

- *Prescription drug management*
- *Decision regarding minor surgery*
  (with identified patient or procedure risk factors)
- *Decision regarding elective major surgery without identified patient or procedure risk factors*
- *Diagnosis or treatment significantly limited by social determinants of health*

High complexity   *High risk of morbidity from additional diagnostic testing or treatment*

Examples only

- *Drug therapy requiring intensive monitoring for toxicity*
- *Decision for elective major surgery with identified patient or procedure risk factors*
- *Decision for emergency major surgery*
- *Decision regarding hospitalization*
- *Decision for DNR or to de-escalate care because of poor prognosis*
- *Parenteral controlled substances*

Source: American Medical Association, 2022

Table 4.18 Subjective, objective, assessment, plan (SOAP) note template: Acute visit

Chief complaint(CC)		What brought you here today?	Short in patient's own words eg. "I have a headache"
History of present illness (HPI)		Chronological order of events, before onset of CC, must include OLDCARTS in paragraph form **INCLUDE SYSTEMIC SYMPTOMS, IS CONDITION IMPROVING, WORSENING, OR UNCHANGED; Chronic illnesses that may be affecting conditions such as COPD**	
	Onset		
	Location		
	Duration		
	Character		
	Aggravating/associated factors		
	Relieving factors		
	Temporal factors – other things going on		
	Severity		
Past medical history		Include if it is at treatment goal or not: Example HTN is at goal of treatment BP < 140/90	
Family hx		Pertinent to CC	

Social hx	Pertinent or needs to be considered eg. in MDM. Examples: Occupational hazard, daycare, smoking, drinking, recreational or illicit drug use	
Allergies		
Medications	Include herbs and over the counter medications	
Review of systems (ROS)	General	
Subjective data You ask questions to uncover more detail; patient confirms or denies symptoms	Hair, skin, & nails	
	Head	
	Neck	
	Eyes	
	Ears	
	Nose	
	Mouth & throat	

(Continued)

Table 4.18 (Continued)

	Cardiovascular	
	Respiratory	
	Breasts	
	Gastrointestinal	
	Musculoskeletal	
	Peripheral	
	Neurological	
	Psychiatric	
Vital signs (VS)	BP P R T pulse oximetry Height Weight BMI	
Physical exam (PE) – Objective data you examine or observe	General	
	Hair, skin, & nails	
	Head	
	Neck	

	Eyes
	Ears
	Nose
	Mouth & throat
	Cardiovascular
	Respiratory
	Breasts
	Gastrointestinal
	Musculoskeletal
	Peripheral
	Neurological
	Psychiatric
Labs reviewed	*Include creatine clearance if known for medication dosing*
Radiology reviewed	
Independent interpretations	*Include if you independently interpreted the results (EKG, CXR) unless this will be billed separately elsewhere such as by radiology*
Differential diagnosis/ plan	*List in rank order with symptoms that support it as well as what tests you will do to rule in/out* 1 2 3

(Continued)

Table 4.18 (Continued)

Diagnosis/plan	Rank order if more than 1 and include your plan – tests, medications etc.
Education/follow up	What will you educate patient on and when do you want them to follow up?
External records reviewed	Did you review records outside of your practice for this encounter? Labs/tests/other provider notes?
Independent historian	Did you obtain information regarding history from someone other than the patient due to mental status, age, or condition to help you in MDM?
Collaboration	Discussion of management with external clinicians or appropriate source
Shared decision making	Testing or treatment considered, even if not done
Social determinants of health	Conditions that may influence patient's conditions (inability to fill prescriptions, transportation, insufficient insurance)
Decision to hospitalize	If considered, state why or why not?
Code status	Decision to de-escalate care because of poor prognosis patient/family wishes

Table 4.19 SOAP note template: Chronic disease management visit

Chief complaint (CC)	What brought you here today?	Short: in patient's own words eg. "I have a headache"
History of present illness (HPI)	Chronological order of events, before onset of CC, must include OLDCARTS in paragraph form INCLUDE SYSTEMIC SYMPTOMS, IS CONDITION IMPROVING, WORSENING, OR UNCHANGED; Chronic illnesses that may be affecting conditions such as COPD	
	Onset	
	Location	
	Duration	
	Character	
	Aggravating/associated factors	
	Relieving factors	
	Temporal factors – other things going on	
	Severity	
Past medical history	Include if it is at treatment goal or not: Example HTN is at goal of treatment BP < 140/90	
Family hx	That is pertinent to CC	
Social hX	That is pertinent or needs to be considered eg. Occupational hazard, daycare, smoking, drinking, recreational or illicit drug use	

(Continued)

Table 4.19 (Continued)

Allergies		
Medications	Include herbs and over the counter medications	
Review of systems (ROS)	General	
	Hair, skin, & nails	
Subjective data	Head	
You ask questions	Neck	
to uncover more	Eyes	
detail patient	Ears	
confirms or denies	Nose	
	Mouth & throat	
	Cardiovascular	
	Respiratory	
	Breasts	
	Gastrointestinal	
	Musculoskeletal	
	Peripheral	
	Neurological	
	Psychiatric	
Vital signs (VS)	BP P R T pulse, oximetry, height, weight, BMI	

Physical exam (PE) – objective data you examine or observe	General	
	Hair, skin, & nails	
	Head	
	Neck	
	Eyes	
	Ears	
	Nose	
	Mouth & throat	
	Cardiovascular	
	Respiratory	
	Breasts	
	Gastrointestinal	
	Musculoskeletal	
	Peripheral	
	Neurological	
	Psychiatric	
Labs reviewed	Include creatine clearance if known for medication dosing	
Radiology reviewed		
Independent interpretations	Include if you independently interpreted the results (EKG, CXR), do not include if it will be billed somewhere else	

(Continued)

Table 4.19 (Continued)

Chronic disease(s)	List in rank order/list plan such as future tests, medications	1 2 3
Education/follow up	What will you educate the patient about and when should they follow up?	
External records reviewed	Did you review records outside of your practice for this encounter? Labs/tests/ other provider notes?	
Independent historian	Did you obtain information regarding history from someone other than the patient due to mental status, age, or condition to help you in MDM?	
Collaboration	Discussion of management with external clinicians or appropriate source	
Shared decision making	Testing or treatment considered, even if not done	
Social determinants of health	Conditions that may influence patient's conditions (inability to fill prescriptions, transportation, insufficient insurance)	
Decision to hospitalize	If considered give reason why or why not	
Code status	Decision to de-escalate care because of poor prognosis patient/family wishes	

Table 4.20 Example with billing code: Acute care office visit

Chief complaint (CC)	What brought you here today? (Short in patient's own words e.g. "I have a headache")	"My throat hurts"
History of present illness (HPI) •	Chronological order of events, before onset of CC, must include OLDCARTS in paragraph form **INCLUDE SYSTEMIC SYMPTOMS, IS CONDITION IMPROVING, WORSENING, OR UNCHANGED; Chronic illnesses that may be affecting conditions such as COPD**	
	Onset	35 yo female went to Jamaica with her husband for vacation and on 4th day there began having a sore throat, she had fever and chills all night but did not have a thermometer. States she felt hot to touch. States pain in throat is progressive, she vomited, and today it is hard for her to swallow.
	Location	
	Duration	
	Character	
	Aggravating/associated factors	
	Relieving factors	No PMH that is significant.
	Temporal factors – other things going on	Pt does not drink, smoke, or use recreational or illicit drugs
	Severity	
Past medical history	Include if it is at treatment goal or not: Example HTN is at goal of treatment BP < 140/90	
Family hx	That is pertinent to CC	
Social hx	That is pertinent or needs to be considered eg., Occupational hazard, daycare, smoking, drinking, recreational or illicit drug use	

(Continued)

Table 4.20 (Continued)

Allergies	NKA	
Medications	Include herbs and over the counter medications	She has Mirena for birth control.
Review of systems (ROS)	Questions you ask to uncover more symptoms related to chief complaint that patient will confirm or deny (pt c/o or pt. denies) to help you come up with differential diagnosis	
	General	Reports feeling feverish, hot, sweaty
	Hair, skin, & nails	
	Head	
	Neck	Denies neck stiffness
	Eyes	Denies photophobia
	Ears	
	Nose	
	Mouth & throat	Pain in throat and neck
	Cardiovascular	Denies chest pain
	Respiratory	Denies shortness of breath
	Breasts	
	Gastrointestinal	Reports nausea with vomiting x1; denies diarrhea
	Musculoskeletal	
	Peripheral	
	Neurological	Denies syncope
	Psychiatric	

Vital signs (VS)	BP P R T pulse, oximetry, height, weight, BMI 138/80 88 16 101.6 5'4" 146 pounds	
Physical exam **(PE) – Objective data** **you examine or** **observe**	General	Well-groomed female appears apprehensive
	Hair, skin, & nails	
	Head	
	Neck	Appears swollen exteriorly more on the left side
	Eyes	
	Ears	
	Nose	Clear no drainage; no sinus tenderness
	Mouth & throat	Uvular displacement to the left, tonsils kissing with exudate and erythema, "hot potato" voice
	Cardiovascular	SR – no murmurs or rubs
	Respiratory	CTA bilaterally
	Breasts	
	Gastrointestinal	Soft, nontender with normal bowel sounds
	Musculoskeletal	
	Peripheral	
	Neurological	Alert x3
	Psychiatric	
Labs	Include creatine clearance if known for medication dosing	Ordered Strep rapid. Ordered Mono spot.

(Continued)

Table 4.20 (Continued)

Radiology		
Independent interpretations	Include if you independently interpreted the results (EKG, CXR)	
Differential diagnosis/plan	List in rank order with symptoms that support it as well as what tests you will do to rule in /out	1 Possible Strep throat as evidenced by physical exam 2 Possible Mono as evidenced by physical exam 3 Probable Peritonsillar abscess uvular displacement – kissing tonsils and hot potato voice
Diagnosis/plan	Rank order if more than 1	1. Mono – confirmed by Mono Spot 2. Possible peritonsillar abscess – send to ER for CT of neck with contrast
Education/follow up	To go to ER for evaluation	
External records reviewed	Did you review records outside of your practice for this encounter? Labs/tests/other provider notes?	No
Independent historian	Did you obtain information regarding history from someone other than the patient due to mental status, age, or condition to help you in MDM?	No

Collaboration	Discussion of management with external clinicians or appropriate source	Discussed with ER physician my findings and sending to ER for further evaluation and management due to nature of probably peritonsillar abscess and escalation of care
Shared decision making	Testing or treatment considered, even if not done	Discussed pros and cons with patient and husband of complications from peritonsillar abscess and airway compromise and decision made to go to ER for further management.
Social determinants of health	Conditions that may influence patient's conditions (inability to fill prescriptions, transportation, insufficient insurance)	Pt has insurance, husband is with her, and they have transportation
Decision to hospitalize	Give reason why or why not	Yes, peritonsillar abscess suspected in presence of Mono coupled with PE findings – decision to hospitalize or not will be made by the ER after evaluation
Code status	Decision to de-escalate care because of poor prognosis patient/family wishes	Full code
Time spent in encounter	This includes all time on this encounter in 24-hour period – face to face and non-face to face time	Total time spent in review of records, examination of patient, ordering testing, interpreting tests, speaking to patient and family regarding decision to go to ER with pros and cons explored, call placed to ER to coordinate care between myself, and ER physician was 45 minutes.

Table 4.21 Calculate the level of care

MDM (Based on 2 out of 3 elements of MDM)	COPA	DATA	RISK
99211	N/A	N/A	N/A
Straight forward 99202 99212 99221 99231 99234	1 self-limited or minor problem	Minimal or NONE	Minimal risk of morbidity from additional diagnostic testing or treatment
Low complexity 99203 99213 99221 99231 99234	2 or more self-limited or minor problems or 1 stable, chronic illness or 1 acute uncomplicated illness or injury or 1 stable, acute illness or 1 acute, uncomplicated illness or injury requiring hospital inpatient or observation level of care	*(Must meet 1 of 2 requirements)* **Category 1: Tests and documents.** *Any combination of 2 from the following* • *Review of prior external note(s) from each unique source* • *Review of the result(s) of each unique test* • *Ordering of each unique test* or **Category 2: Assessment requiring an independent historian(s)**	Low risk of morbidity from additional diagnostic testing or treatment

| **Moderate**
99204
99214
99222
99232
99235 | 1 or more chronic illnesses with exacerbation, progression, or side effects of treatment

or

2 or more stable chronic illnesses

or

1 undiagnosed new problem with uncertain prognosis

or

1 acute illness with systemic symptoms

or

1 acute, complicated injury | *(Must meet 1 out of 3 requirements)*
Category 1: Tests, documents, historian
Any combination of 3 from the following

• Review of prior external note(s) from each unique source
• Review of the result(s) of each unique test
• Ordering of each unique test
• Assessment requiring an independent historian(s)

or

Category 2: Independent interpretation of tests

• Independent interpretation of a test performed by another physician/other qualified healthcare professional not separately reported)

or

Category 3: Discussion of management or test interpretation

• Discussion of management or test interpretation with external/physician/other qualified healthcare professional/ appropriate source (not separately reported) | *Moderate risk of morbidity from additional diagnostic testing or treatment*
Examples only:

• Prescription drug management
• Decision regarding minor surgery (with identified patient or procedure risk factors)
• Decision regarding elective major surgery (without identified patient or procedure risk factors)
• Diagnosis or treatment significantly limited by social determinants of health |

(Continued)

Table 4.21 (Continued)

MDM (Based on 2 out of 3 elements of MDM)	COPA	DATA	RISK
High complexity 99205 99215 99223 99233 99236	1 or more chronic illnesses with severe exacerbation, progression, or side effects of treatment or 1 acute or chronic illness or injury that poses a threat to life or bodily function or Multiple morbidities requiring intensive management (Initial Nursing Facility only)	*(Must meet 2 out of 3 requirements)* **Category 1: Tests, documents, historian** *Any combination of 3 from the following* • Review of prior external note(s) from each unique source • Review of the result(s) of each unique test • Ordering of each unique test • Assessment requiring an independent historian(s) or **Category 2: Independent interpretation of tests** • Independent interpretation of a test performed by another physician/other qualified healthcare professional (not separately reported) or **Category 3: Discussion of management or test interpretation** • Discussion of management or test interpretation with external/physician/other qualified healthcare professional/appropriate source (not separately reported)	High risk of morbidity from additional diagnostic testing or treatment Examples only: • Drug therapy requiring intensive monitoring for toxicity • Decision for elective major surgery with identified patient or procedure risk factors • Decision for emergency major surgery • Decision regarding hospitalization • Decision for DNR or to de-escalate care because of poor prognosis • Parenteral controlled substances

Table 4.22 Summary of level of care

MDM	COPA	DATA	RISK
Moderate		Discussion of management or test interpretation with external/physician/ other qualified healthcare professional/appropriate source (not separately reported)	
High	1 acute or chronic illness or injury that poses a threat to life or bodily function		Decision regarding hospitalization
Time	45 minutes		

Table 4.23 Reimbursement rates for established office visits

Established office visit					2023 rates
E/M code	History	Exam	MDM (2 out of 3)	Time	Reimbursement
99211	History and physical exam should be appropriate as determined by the physician and no longer is calculated into billing		None	NA	$23.38*
99212			Straightforward	10–19	$56.93*
99213			Low complexity	20–29	$90.82*
99214			Mod complexity	30–39	$128.43*
99215			High complexity	40–54	$179.94*

* Rates are from the AMA based on 2023 prices

MDM = 99215 High

Time = 99215 High

Table 4-24 Example: Chronic office visit

Chief complaint (CC)		What brought you here today? (Short in patient's own words eg. "I have a headache")	"My blood sugars are really low at times"
History of present illness (HPI)		Chronological order of events, before onset of CC, must include OLDCARTS in paragraph form INCLUDE SYSTEMIC SYMPTOMS, IS CONDITION IMPROVING, WORSENING, OR UNCHANGED; Chronic illnesses that may be affecting conditions such as COPD	68 yo male lives alone, h/o dementia and type 2 diabetes has had several episodes of feeling faint and when blood sugars were checked they were between 40–60 per the patients' blood sugar log, however other blood sugars before lunch and dinner indicate high readings between 250–350. Daughter reports that her father may not be checking his blood sugars at the correct time, and family friend who checks on the patient regularly is not sure he is dosing the insulin correctly. Symptoms are relieved when he eats food.
	Onset		
	Location		
	Duration		
	Character		
	Aggravating/associated factors		
	Relieving factors		
	Temporal factors – other things going on		
	Severity		
Past medical history		Include if it is at treatment goal or not: Example HTN is at goal of treatment BP < 140/90	Dementia
Family hx		That is pertinent to CC	
Social hx		That is pertinent or needs to be considered eg. Occupational hazard, daycare, smoking, drinking, recreational or illicit drug use	Pt smokes 1 ppd of cigarettes and has for the past 40 years

Allergies	NKA	
Medications	Include herbs and over the counter medications	Metformin 500mg BID/Levemir 20 units at HS
Review of systems (ROS)	Questions you ask to uncover more symptoms related to chief complaint that patient will confirm or deny (pt c/o or pt denies) to help you come up with differential diagnosis	
	General	Has not lost weight or gained weight
	Hair, skin, & nails	
	Head	
	Neck	
	Eyes	
	Ears	
	Nose	
	Mouth & throat	
	Cardiovascular	No c/o chest pain
	Respiratory	No c/o shortness of breath
	Breasts	
	Gastrointestinal	No c/o diarrhea or change in color of stool
	Musculoskeletal	
	Peripheral	
	Neurological	c/o feeling light-headed at times like he is going to pass out, feels sweaty
	Psychiatric	Daughter reports he has been a little more confused lately

(Continued)

Table 4-24 (Continued)

Vital signs (VS)		BP P R T pulse, oximetry, height, weight, BMI
		120/80 88 16 98.6 5'5 155
Physical exam (PE) – Objective data you examine or observe	General	Ill kept elderly gentleman older than stated age
	Hair, skin, & nails	
	Head	
	Neck	
	Eyes	
	Ears	
	Nose	
	Mouth & throat	Caries present
	Cardiovascular	Normal sinus rhythm with no murmurs clicks or rubs
	Respiratory	CTA bilaterally
	Breasts	
	Gastrointestinal	Soft, nontender with normal bowel sounds
	Musculoskeletal	
	Peripheral	
	Neurological	Cranial nerves II-XII grossly intact
	Psychiatric	Alert x3 answers questions appropriately

Labs	Include creatine clearance if known for medication dosing	Reviewed the last hemoglobin A1c when he was in hospital 1 month ago from hospital records and it was 7.5
Radiology		None
Independent interpretations	Include if you independently interpreted the results (EKG, CXR)	Reviewed blood sugar logs – AM blood sugars usually under 100 lowest 40 (twice in last week) – rest of blood sugars between 250–350
Chronic disease(s)	List in rank order/list plan	Diabetes Mellitus – type 2 – adjust insulin back to previous dose of 15 units/monitor blood sugar logs – return in 1 week. Dementia – possible exacerbation – daughter will come to home and give patient insulin at correct times to make sure it is done correctly and check blood sugars
Education/follow up: daughter to call office in 1 week with logs AC and HS x 1 week for further adjustments		
External records reviewed	Did you review records outside of your practice for this encounter? Labs/tests/other provider notes?	Yes, hospital records reviewed with discharge medication changes noted
Independent historian	Did you obtain information regarding history from someone other than the patient due to mental status, age, or condition to help you in MDM?	Yes, obtained information from daughter who verified patient may not be checking blood sugars correctly or dosing insulin correctly as he has been more confused lately

(Continued)

Table 4-24 (Continued)

Collaboration	Discussion of management with external clinicians or appropriate source	No
Shared decision making	Testing or treatment considered, even if not done	Discussed tolerance of hemoglobin A1c at higher levels due to his age and mental status with risk factors of hypoglycemia being greater since he lives alone. Decision made to tolerate a higher hemoglobin A1c of 7.5 or below to avoid hypoglycemic events.
Social determinants of health	Conditions that may influence patient's conditions (inability to fill prescriptions, transportation, insufficient insurance)	Pt does not have any social determinants of health that would influence care/he has adequate insurance and family support.
Decision to hospitalize	Give reason why or why not	No

Code status	Decision to de-escalate care because of poor prognosis patient/family wishes	Pt is a Full code
Time spent in encounter	This includes all time on this encounter in 24-hour period – face to face and non-face to face time	60 minutes spent in review of record, examination of patient, discussion with daughter in regards to patient's memory and recent events, shared decision making was discussed in regards to diabetic management and risk of hypoglycemia, plan was developed for daughter to go to father's home and give insulin before meals and at bedtime as well as keep a log of blood sugars obtained, insulin is adjusted down and will be titrated further based on results of blood sugars. Daughter to call office in 1 week and give BS log and report on how patient is doing. Documentation was completed and future tests and medications ordered.

Table 4.25 Calculate the level of care

MDM (Based on 2 out of 3 elements of MDM)	Number of problems	Complexity of data reviewed	Risk of complications and or morbidity
99211	N/A	N/A	N/A
Straightforward 99202 99212 99221 99231 99234	1 self-limited or minor problem	Minimal or NONE	Minimal risk of morbidity from additional diagnostic testing or treatment
Low complexity 99203 99213 99221 99231 99234	2 or more self-limited or minor problems **or** 1 stable, chronic illness **or** 1 acute uncomplicated illness or injury **or** 1 stable, acute illness	(Must meet 1 of 2 requirements) **Category 1: Tests and documents** Any combination of 2 from the following • Review of prior external note(s) from each unique source • Review of the result(s) of each unique test • Ordering of each unique test	Low risk of morbidity from additional diagnostic testing or treatment

Moderate		or	
99204	1 or more chronic illnesses with exacerbation, progression, or side effects of treatment	1 acute, uncomplicated illness or injury requiring hospital inpatient or observation level of care	Moderate risk of morbidity from additional diagnostic testing or treatment
99214			
99222		**Category 2: Assessment requiring an independent historian(s)**	Examples only:
99232	or		
99235	2 or more stable chronic illnesses	(Must meet 1 out of 3 requirements)	*Prescription drug management*
	or	**Category 1: Tests, documents, historian**	
	1 undiagnosed new problem with uncertain prognosis	Any combination of 3 from the following	• Decision regarding minor surgery
		• Review of prior external note(s) from each unique source	• with identified patient or procedure risk factors
	or	• Review of the result(s) of each unique test	• Decision regarding elective major surgery without identified patient or procedure risk factors
	1 acute illness with systemic symptoms	• Ordering of each unique test	
	or	• Assessment requiring an independent historian(s)	• Diagnosis or treatment significantly limited by social determinants of health
	1 acute, complicated injury	or	
		Category 2: Independent interpretation of tests	
		• Independent interpretation of a test performed by another physician/other qualified healthcare professional (not separately reported)	

(Continued)

Table 4-25 (Continued)

MDM (Based on 2 out of 3 elements of MDM)	Number of problems	Complexity of data reviewed	Risk of complications and or morbidity
		or	
		Category 3: Discussion of management or test interpretation	
		• *Discussion of management or test interpretation with external/ physician/other qualified healthcare professional/ appropriate source (not separately reported)*	
High complexity 99205 99215 99223 99233 99236	*1 or more chronic illnesses with severe exacerbation, progression, or side effects of treatment* **or** *1 acute or chronic illness or injury that poses a threat to life or bodily function* **or** *Multiple morbidities requiring intensive management (Initial Nursing Facility only)*	*(Must meet 2 out of 3 requirements)* **Category 1: Tests, documents, historian** *Any combination of 3 from the following* • *Review of prior external note(s) from each unique source* • *Review of the result(s) of each unique test* • *Ordering of each unique test* • *Assessment requiring an independent historian(s)*	*High risk of morbidity from additional diagnostic testing or treatment* Examples only: • *Drug therapy requiring intensive monitoring for toxicity* • *Decision for elective major surgery with identified patient or procedure risk factors*

or

Category 2: Independent interpretation of tests

- *Independent interpretation of a test performed by another physician / other qualified healthcare professional (not separately reported)*

or

Category 3: Discussion of management or test interpretation

- *Discussion of management or test interpretation with external / physician / other qualified healthcare professional / appropriate source (not separately reported)*

- *Decision for emergency major surgery*
- *Decision regarding hospitalization*
- *Decision for DNR or to de-escalate care because of poor prognosis*
- *Parenteral controlled substances*

Table 4.26 Summary of the level of care

MDM	COPA	DATA	RISK
SF			
Low			
Moderate	1 or more chronic illnesses with exacerbation, progression, or side effects of treatment	• Review of prior external note(s) from each unique source • Review of the result(s) of each unique test • Ordering of each unique test • Assessment requiring an independent historian(s)	• Prescription drug-management
High			
Time	60 minutes		

Table 4.27 Reimbursement rates for established office visits

Established office visit					*2023 rates
E/M Code	History	Exam	MDM (2 out of 3)	Time	Reimbursement
99211	History and physical exam should be appropriate as determined by the physician and no longer is calculated into billing		None	NA	$24*
99212			Straightforward	10–19	$57*
99213			Low Complexity	20–29	$92*
99214			Mod Complexity	30–39	$130*
99215			High Complexity	40–54	$183*

Source: Centers for Medicare and Medicaid Services [CMS], 2023

* Rates are from the AMA based on 2023 prices

MDM = 99214 Moderate

Time = 99215 High

Using the MDM tool this patient had 3 out of 3 in the Moderate level and only needed 2 out of 3 to qualify for that level. Using the established office patient level of service code that would be a 99214. However, time was documented as 60 minutes and documentation was detailed to include information on reviewing records, examining patient, discussing care management with daughter and patient with options under shared decision making as well as a follow up plan, documentation and ordering of future labs and medications so a 99215 is justified using time as our indicator (American Medical Association, 2022).

TIME

Under the new 2023 guidelines you can use the MDM tool or time whichever gives you the greater reimbursement. Each category of service has different time codes, so it is important to review the time codes for your specialty (refer to Chapter 6). Note that the ER does **NOT** allow time to be a descriptive component because of the nature of that visit being so variable. According to the 2023 rules time now includes face-to-face time **AND** non-face-to-face time on the day of service (24 hours) which includes the following:

- Review of tests/record *prior to seeing the patient*
- The *interview/physical exam* portion of seeing the patient
- *Counseling or educating* the patient/family/or caregiver
- *Ordering medications/tests or procedures*
- Referring and communicating with other healthcare professionals (not separately reported)
- Documenting the encounter
- Independently interpreting results (not separately reported) and communicating results to the patient/family or caregiver
- Coordination of care

(American Medical Association, 2022)

In our chronic care example, you can see where the provider had a patient who had dementia, which prompted more time and investigation into the home situation with the daughter, shared decision making was done in addition to the normal review of the record and examination of the patient. A follow-up plan to reevaluate the patient's blood sugars and make any further adjustments to medication was documented as well as finalization of the note and ordering of medications and future testing. This was well documented and justified the 60-minute office visit.

Another example might be non-continuous time in the event you saw a patient in the morning and spent 10 minutes reviewing the record prior to seeing the patient and then spent 20 minutes examining the patient and ordering tests. The patient goes home, you still need to complete the documentation and while doing this see the lab results come in. You note the hemoglobin is dangerously low and the patient needs to go to the hospital for a transfusion. You call the patient and tell them they need to go to the local emergency room as well as call the ER and tell the doctor in the ER the situation. You then document this interaction as well as complete all your documentation for the encounter. Under the 2023 guidelines you can count all that time (during the day of the visit) if you document it. Prior to 2023 you could only count the face-to-face time.

One caveat to consider when billing for time is you can **NOT** bill for more time than is in a day, for example if you have billed for 1 hour of service for 26 patients in a day you will be liable for fraudulent billing if caught. Be sure to be accurate and thorough to get paid what you should be paid for your medical decision making and no more.

REFERENCES

AAPC Thought Leadership Team. (2024, June 27). *E/m coding for outpatient services*. AAPC. Retrieved September 18, 2024, from https://www.aapc.com/resources/evaluation-management-coding-outpatient-services

American Medical Association. (2022). *CPT 2022 professional edition*. American Medical Association.

Centers for Medicare and Medicaid Services. (2023). *Search the physician fee schedule*. https://www.cms.gov/medicare/physician-fee-schedule/search

SPECIALTY SERVICES

PSYCHIATRIC SERVICES

Psychiatric services can be performed in several different settings, and prior to the 2023 changes different rules applied to different settings making psychiatric billing very confusing. Office visit and outpatient exams utilized the 2021 MDM tool or time, but all other places of service utilized the E/M 1997 guidelines which had a different psychiatric physical exam as part of the documentation. Every component in the boxes below needed to be present in the note. If the patient was in the ER the type of note depended on whether the patient was discharged or admitted making it more confusing.

With the 2023 rule changes you no longer need to gather a specific psychiatric physical exam, it is up to the provider to conduct an appropriate history and physical exam for the visit which simplifies things considerably. However, that does not mean the provider does not do a thorough assessment. The most important thing for you to remember as a NP is to give an *accurate picture of the patient's story that helps explain your medical decision-making process.*

DOI: 10.4324/9781003542872-5

Example Psychiatric visit – New patient (2023 rules)

CC: "My anxiety is getting worse, and I feel my heart racing."

HPI: 24-year-old female comes in with increasing anxiety for several months. She states

she has always had anxiety, but it is much worse since she and her boyfriend split up. Her primary care provider started her on Prozac about a month ago. She feels as if her heart is racing at times. She recently went to the emergency department because of it, and they gave her metoprolol to slow down her heart. She saw a cardiologist who said everything was okay with her heart, but she continues to have these attacks. She doesn't know what to do to make things better and states it is starting to affect her quality of life.

Medications: Prozac 20mg daily, Metoprolol 25mg XL daily

Fam hx: Mother has h/o depression and anxiety.

Social hx: She does not smoke or drink energy drinks, coffee, or soda, but states she has been drinking more ETOH lately – 2–3 times a week she has 1–3 drinks at night after work.

PE: VS B/P 140/80 P 105 R 16

    General: alert and well-groomed with normal speech

    Resp: lungs clear to auscultation

    Cardiac: Sinus tachycardic – no murmurs, thrills, or rubs noted

    Skin: warm and dry, color pale

    Psychiatric: normal thought process with abstract reasoning, denies suicidal or homicidal ideation, has good insight and appropriate judgment, good attention span with normal mood and affect.

ASSESSMENT/PLAN:

- Increase Prozac to 40mg daily.
- Reviewed ER record and cardiologist notes. Echocardiogram was normal and TSH panel was normal.
- Ordered Vitamin D level.
- Referral to behavioral counseling.
- Hydroxyzine 25mg TID prn prescribed.

Table 5.1 Psychiatric physical exam conducted to 1997 guidelines

Psychiatric Physical Exam per 1997 guidelines

Constitutional	• *Measurement of any three of the following seven VS 1.) sitting or standing BP 2.) supine BP, 3.) Pulse rate and regularity 4.) respirations 5.) temperature 6.) height, or 7.) weight (this may be measured and recorded by ancillary staff)* • *General appearance of patient (eg. development, nutrition, body habitus, deformities, attention to grooming)*
Musculoskeletal	• *Assessment of muscle strength and tone (eg. Flaccid, cog wheel, spastic) with notation of any atrophy and abnormal movements* • *Examination of gait and station*

Psychiatric	• *Description of speech including rate, volume, articulation, coherence, and spontaneity with notation of abnormalities (eg. preservation, paucity of language)*
	• *Description of thought processes including rate of thoughts, content of thoughts (eg. logical vs illogical, tangential) abstract reasoning, and computation*
	• *Description of associations (eg. loose, tangential, circumstantial, intact)*
	• *Description of abnormal or psychotic thoughts including hallucinations; delusions; preoccupation with violence, homicidal or suicidal ideations, and obsessions*
	• *Description of the patient's judgment (eg. concerning everyday activities and social situations) and insight (eg. concerning psychiatric conditions)*
	• *Complete mental status examination including:*
	  • *Orientation to time, place and person*
	  • *Recent and remote memory*
	  • *Attention span and concentrations*
	  • *Language (eg. naming objects, repeating phrases)*
	  • *Fund of knowledge (eg. awareness of current events, past history, vocabulary)*
	  • *Mood and effect (eg. depression, anxiety, agitation, hypomania, lability)*

Total visit was 45 minutes including face-to-face time including calculating a generalized anxiety disorder (GAD) score and depression score, with physical exam and ordering medication, tests, and follow up. Since this is an initial exam, you would use one of the following codes:

A 90791 is an integrated biopsychosocial assessment, that includes history, mental status, and recommendations. It may also include communication with a friend, or family member, and is usually used by a therapist.

A 90792 is the appropriate code for this visit because it includes a psychiatric diagnostic evaluation **WITH** medical services and includes an integrated biopsychosocial **and medical assessment**, including history, mental status, and other physical examination elements as indicated. *This is the code that most providers will use* (psychiatrists, NPs). For subsequent visits they will use the normal E/M billing codes for 2023 established office visits (99212–99215).

Table 5.2 Initial exam codes

90791	*Psychiatric diagnostic evaluation*
90792	*Psychiatric diagnostic evaluation with medical services*

CLINICAL PEARL

On subsequent visits do NOT chart things like *"patient is doing well no change in plan."* When an insurance carrier or auditor is reading that note they do not have access to your previous notes without requesting them, be sure and explain what you mean by *doing well* and ask yourself, if they are doing well enough, do they need to continue to see you so often? Are they stable enough to transition to their primary caregiver? If you are continuing to need to see them more frequently be sure and explain this in your documentation.

CONSULTATIONS

Consult services are made when a provider requests another provider for an opinion for a specific problem that the consulting provider has expertise in. For example, if your patient has a complicated heart problem you may consult a cardiologist to see them. This can occur in both the inpatient and outpatient worlds. The consulting provider should provide a written report to the consulting physician.

Prior to 2023 changes this was again a very complicated process. The 2023 changes have simplified this considerably and now there are only two sets to consider: either the office/outpatient setting or the inpatient/observation setting.

Table 5.3 E/M 2023 Initial office/other outpatient consultation (for new or established patients)

E/M code	History	Exam	MDM	Time
99242	*History and physical exam should be appropriate as determined by the physician and are longer calculated into billing*		*Straightforward*	*20 minutes*
99243			*Low complexity*	*30 minutes*
99244			*Mod complexity*	*40 minutes*
99245			*High complexity*	*55 minutes*

Subsequent visits should be coded 99212–99215 (established office visit) or home or residence (99347–99350).

Table 5.4 E/M 2023 Initial consultations inpatient/observation/rehab (for new or established patients)

E/M code	History	Exam	MDM	Time
99252	*History and physical exam should be appropriate as determined by the physician and are no longer calculated into billing*		*Straightforward*	*35 minutes*
99253			*Low complexity*	*45 minutes*
99254			*Mod complexity*	*60 minutes*
99255			*High complexity*	*80 minutes*

Subsequent consultations during the same visit should be coded as subsequent inpatient or observation hospital care codes (99231–99233) or subsequent nursing facility care codes (99307–99310).

TELEHEATH VISITS

Telehealth services were expanded greatly during the COVID 19 pandemic to accommodate people staying at home. NP services were broadened as well as the CPT codes you could bill for. The following chart shows the before and after COVID 19 regulations.

Table 5.5 NP services before and after the COVID 19 pandemic

Level	Before COVID 19	After COVID 19
Virtual check-in	• *Established patient* • *Initiated by patient* • *Brief communication with physician in lieu of an in-person visit* • *Pt must provide verbal consent* • *Co-pay does apply* • *Cannot be related to a previous visit within the last 7 days or result in an in-person visit within the next 24 hours* • *Can be phone, audiovisual interface, text, email, patient portal*	• *Can be new or established patient* • *Provider can waive co-pay*
Electronic visits 99421: 5–10 minutes 99422: 11–20 minutes 99423: 21 minutes or more	• *Established patients only* • *Initiated by the patient* • *Text or communication is part of permanent record* • *Online digital E/M through a secure patient portal* • *Co-pay applies* • *Code based on cumulative time over 7-day period*	• *Can be new or established patient* • *Provider can waive co-pay*

| Telephone E/M visits
99441: 5–10 minutes
99442: 11–20 minutes
99443: 21–30 minutes | • Established patients only
• Cannot be used if they are in follow up for a visit within the past 7 days or if they result in a in-person visit within 24 hours | • Can be new or established patient
• Provider can waive co-pay |
| Telehealth visits | • Provided on a limited basis
• Patient must be established
• Patient must be in a rural location
• Patient had to travel to an approved site
• Required use of a HIPAA compliant real-time, two-way audiovisual interface
• Point of service was 02 so it was paid at lower rate than in the office
• Only a few types of services were offered | • Pt and provider can be located anywhere
• New or existing patient
• Visits paid as in-person visit
• Provider can waive co-pay
• Still requires real-time, two-way audiovisual communications
• HIPPAA communication can be waived but must use FACETIME, SKYPE, or ZOOM
• Almost all visits are accepted |

The biggest category to change was the telehealth visit. Post COVID 19, you can bill the same for this visit as if the patient were in your office by attaching a 95 modifier. It is important to note that these rules may revert partially or completely back to prior COVID 19 rules once we are out of this pandemic completely and can vary state by state. At the height of COVID 19 providers from any state could treat patients in any state, but that is gradually reverting to the rule that a provider can only treat patients if they hold a license in that state. Make sure during a telehealth visit you note where the patient is located, such as at home during the visit, and where you, the NP are at, and document this as part of the encounter.

It is also important to realize the opportunity that the pandemic provided for NPs and advanced providers. Due to the high need for medical care all but 7 states limiting APRN practice relaxed their rules by either partially or fully waiving collaborative practice agreements. NPs were allowed to practice to the full extent of their education paving the way for future **national** full practice authority (Stucky et al., 2020).

MEDICARE WELLNESS VISITS

G-0402 Initial Preventive Physical Exam (IPPE) – is known as the *WELCOME TO MEDICARE PREVENTIVE VISIT* – it is only done once and must be performed by one of the following:

- Physician (MD, DO)
- Qualified non-physician practitioner (NP, PA, CNS)

It includes a once in a lifetime EKG that can be ordered at that time.

G-0438 Initial Annual Wellness Exam (AWN) – it is the first exam patients have after turning 65 and must be performed by one of the following:

- Physician (MD, DO)
- Qualified non-physician practitioner (NP, PA, CNS)
- Medical professional such as a health educator, registered dietitian, or other licensed professionals the physician directly supervises.

G-0439 Subsequent AWN must be performed by one of the following:

- Physician (MD, DO)
- Qualified non-physician practitioner (NP, PA, CNS)
- Medical professional such as a health educator, registered dietitian, or other licensed professional the physician directly supervises (American Medical Association, 2022).

REFERENCES

American Medical Association. (2022). *CPT professional 2023 and E/M companion 2023 and CPT quickref app bundle.* American Medical Association Press.

Centers for Medicare and Medicaid Services. (2022, August). *MLN6775421 – Medicare wellness visits.* https://www.cms.gov/Outreach-and-Education/Medicare-Learning-Network-MLN/MLNProducts/preventive-services/medicare-wellness-visits.html

Stucky, C., Brown, W., & Stucky, M. (2021). COVID 19. An unprecedented opportunity for nurse practitioners to reform healthcare and advocate for permanent full practice authority. *Nursing Forum, 56*(1), 222–227. https://doi.org/10.1111/nuf.12515

EXAMPLES OF DOCUMENTATION WITH CODING

Table 6.1 Office visits E/M 2021/2023: new office visit

CC	*Left sided ear pain*
HPI	*6-year-old male comes in with c/o left sided ear pain, that started last night, mother reports he was up most of the night c/o pain, fever was up to 102.6. He could not sleep with it.*
PFSH	*Last ear infection 2 years ago*
ROS	**HEENT**: *c/o left sided ear pain, no c/o sore throat or cold symptoms.* **GI:** *no c/o nausea/vomiting*
PE	**General**: *well developed 6-year-old male, who does not appear to feel well.* **HEENT**: *Left TM bulging with no landmarks, fluid filled, throat without edema, nares patent.* **Lungs**: *CTA* **Cardiac**: *Normal rate and rhythm*
A/P	*Otitis Medica – left – prescribed Augmentin BID for 10 days*
Time	*20 minutes (review of records, examination of patient, discussion with mother, documentation, and preparation of discharge paperwork to include prescription)*

DOI: 10.4324/9781003542872-6

Table 6.2 New office visit E/M codes

E/M code	History/Exam	MDM	Time
99202	*Clinician required to perform and document medically appropriate history and examination*	*Straightforward*	*Or 15–29*
99203		*Low complexity*	*Or 30–44*
99204		*Mod complexity*	*Or 45–59*
99205		*High complexity*	*Or 60–74*

MDM = 99203 Low

Time = 99292 Straightforward

Table 6.3 Medical decision-making tool

MDM (2 out of 3 MDM)	Number of problems	Complexity of data reviewed	Risk of complications and or morbidity
Straightforward 99202 99212 99221 99231 99234	*1 self-limited or minor problem*	*Minimal or NONE*	*Minimal risk of morbidity from additional diagnostic testing or treatment*
Low complexity 99203 99213 99221 99231 99234	*2 or more self-limited or minor problems* *or* *1 stable, chronic illness* *or* *1 acute uncomplicated illness or injury* *or* *1 stable, acute illness* *or* *1 acute, uncomplicated illness or injury requiring hospital inpatient or observation level of care*	*(Must meet 1 of 2 requirements)* **Category 1: Tests and documents** *Any combination of 2 from the following* • *Review of prior external note(s) from each unique source* • *Review of the result(s) of each unique test* • *Ordering of each unique test* OR **Category 2: Assessment requiring an independent historian(s)**	*Low risk of morbidity from additional diagnostic testing or treatment*

| **Moderate**
99204
99214
99222
99232
99235 | *1 or more chronic illnesses with exacerbation, progression, or side effects of treatment*

or

2 or more stable chronic illnesses

or

1 undiagnosed new problem with uncertain prognosis

or

1 acute illness with systemic symptoms

or

1 acute, complicated injury | *(Must meet 1 out of 3 requirements)*
Category 1: Tests, documents, historian
Any combination of 3 from the following
• *Review of prior external note(s) from each unique source*
• *Review of the result(s) of each unique test*
• *Ordering of each unique test*
• *Assessment requiring an independent historian(s)*
OR
Category 2: Independent interpretation of tests
• *Independent interpretation of a test performed by another physician/other qualified healthcare professional (not separately reported).*
OR
Category 3: Discussion of management or test interpretation
• *Discussion of management or test interpretation with external/physician/other qualified healthcare professional/appropriate source (not separately reported)* | *Moderate risk of morbidity from additional diagnostic testing or treatment*
Examples only:
• *Prescription drug management*
• *Decision regarding minor surgery with identfied patient or procedure risk factors*
• *Decision regarding elective major surgery without identified patient or procedure risk factors*
• *Diagnosis or treatment significantly limited by social determinants of health* |

(Continued)

Table 6.3 (Continued)

MDM (2 out of 3 MDM)	Number of problems	Complexity of data reviewed	Risk of complications and or morbidity
High complexity 99205 99215 99223 99233 99236	*1 or more chronic illnesses with severe exacerbation, progression, or side effects of treatment,* **or** *1 acute or chronic illness or injury that poses a threat to life or bodily function* **or** *Multiple morbidities requiring intensive management (Initial Nursing Facility only)*	*(Must meet 2 out of 3 requirements)* **Category 1: Tests, documents, historian** *Any combination of 3 from the following* • *Review of prior external note(s) from each unique source* • *Review of the result(s) of each unique test* • *Ordering of each unique test* • *Assessment requiring an independent historian(s)* **or** **Category 2: Independent interpretation of tests** • *Independent interpretation of a test performed by another physician/other qualified healthcare professional (not separately reported)* **or** **Category 3: Discussion of management or test interpretation** • *Discussion of management or test interpretation with external/physician/ other qualified healthcare professional/appropriate source (not separately reported)*	*High risk of morbidity from additional diagnostic testing or treatment* Examples only: • *Drug therapy requiring intensive monitoring for toxicity* • *Decision for elective major surgery with identified patient or procedure risk factors* • *Decision for emergency major surgery* • *Decision regarding hospitalization* • *Decision for DNR or to de-escalate care because of poor prognosis* • *Parenteral controlled substances*

Table 6.4 Office visits E/M 2021/2023: established office visit

CC	*Let sided ear pain*
HPI	*6-year-old male comes in with c/o left sided ear pain, that stated last night, mother reports he was up most of the night c/o pain, fever was up to 102.6. He could not sleep with it.*
PFSH	*Last ear infection 2 years ago*
ROS	**HEENT**: *c/o left sided ear pain, no c/o sore throat or cold symptoms*
	GI: *no c/o nausea/vomiting*
PE	**General**: *well-developed 6-year-old male, who does not appear to feel well*
	HEENT: *Left TM bulging with no landmarks, fluid filled, throat without edema, nares patent*
	Lungs: *CTA*
	Cardiac: *Normal rate and rhythm*
A/P	*Otitis Medica – left – prescribed Augmentin BID for 10 days*
Time	*20 minutes (review of records, examination of patient, discussion with mother, documentation, and preparation of discharge paperwork to include prescription)*

Note this is exact same note as the NEW patient, but TIME requirements are different for the new and established office visit rates.

Table 6.5 Established office visit E/M codes

E/M code	History/Exam	MDM	Time
99211	*Clinician required to perform and document medically appropriate history and examination*	*None*	*NA*
99212		*Straightforward*	*Or 10–19*
99213		*Low complexity*	*Or 20–29*
99214		*Mod complexity*	*Or 30–39*
99215		*High complexity*	*Or 40–54*

MDM = 99213 Low

Time = 99213 Low

Table 6.6 Medical decision-making tool

MDM (2 out of 3 MDM)	Number of problems	Complexity of data reviewed	Risk of complications and or morbidity
Straight forward 99202 99212 99221 99231 99234	*1 self-limited or minor problem*	*Minimal or NONE*	*Minimal risk of morbidity from additional diagnostic testing or treatment*
Low complexity 99203 99213 99221 99231 99234	*2 or more self-limited or minor problems,* **or** *1 stable, chronic illness,* **or** *1 acute uncomplicated illness or injury* **or** *1 stable, acute illness* **or** *1 acute, uncomplicated illness or injury requiring hospital inpatient or observation level of care*	*(Must meet 1 of 2 requirements)* **Category 1: Tests and documents** *Any combination of 2 from the following* • *Review of prior external note(s) from each unique source* • *Review of the result(s) of each unique test* • *Ordering of each unique test* **or** **Category 2: Assessment requiring an independent historian(s)**	*Low risk of morbidity from additional diagnostic testing or treatment*

| **Moderate**
99204
99214
99222
99232
99235 | 1 or more chronic illnesses with exacerbation, progression, or side effects of treatment

or

2 or more stable chronic illnesses

or

1 undiagnosed new problem with uncertain prognosis

or

1 acute illness with systemic symptoms

or

1 acute, complicated injury | *(Must meet requirements of 1 out of 3)*
Category 1: Tests, documents, historian
Any combination of 3 from the following
• Review of prior external note(s) from each unique source
• Review of the results (s) of each unique test
• Ordering of each unique test
• Assessment requiring an independent historian(s)

or

Category 2: Independent interpretation of tests
• Independent interpretation of a test performed by another physician/other qualified healthcare professional (not separately reported)

or

Category 3: Discussion of management or test interpretation.
• Discussion of management or test interpretation with external/physician/other qualified healthcare professional/appropriate source (not separately reported) | *Moderate risk of morbidity from additional diagnostic testing or treatment*
Examples only:

• *Prescription drug management*
• *Decision regarding minor surgery with identified patient or procedure risk factors*
• *Decision regarding elective major surgery without identified patient or procedure risk factors.*
• *Diagnosis or treatment significantly limited by social determinants of health* |

(Continued)

Table 6.6 (Continued)

MDM (2 out of 3 MDM)	Number of problems	Complexity of data reviewed	Risk of complications and or morbidity
High complexity 99205 99215 99223 99233 99236	*1 or more chronic illnesses with severe exacerbation, progression, or side effects of treatment* **or** *1 acute or chronic illness or injury that poses a threat to life or bodily function* **or** *Multiple morbidities requiring intensive management (Initial Nursing Facility only)*	*(Must meet 2 out of 3 requirements of)* **Category 1: Tests, documents, historian** *Any combination of 3 from the following* • *Review of prior external note(s) from each unique source* • *Review of the result(s) of each unique test* • *Ordering of each unique test* • *Assessment requiring an independent historian(s)* **Category 2: Independent interpretation of tests** • *Independent interpretation of a test performed by another physician/other qualified healthcare professional (not separately reported)* **or** **Category 3: Discussion of management or test interpretation** • *Discussion of management or test interpretation with external/physician/other qualified healthcare professional/appropriate source (not separately reported)*	*High risk of morbidity from additional diagnostic testing or treatment* Examples only: • *Drug therapy requiring intensive monitoring for toxicity.* • *Decision for elective major surgery with identified patient or procedure risk factors* • *Decision for emergency major surgery* • *Decision regarding hospitalization* • *Decision for DNR or to de-escalate care because of poor prognosis.* • *Parenteral controlled substances*

Table 6.7 Inpatient or initial observation: acute care

CC	*Altered mental status*
HPI	*76-year-old female who lives alone in independent living, found by son confused in the bathroom covered with feces. States he and his mother went out to lunch earlier. She was completely normal for that time. States she had recently been diagnosed with shingles and was started on some new medication, but he does not know the name of it. He is unaware if she had any previous kidney problems.*
PFSH	*h/o stroke in past with residual left sided weakness*
ROS	*Unable to obtain due to mental status − refer to HPI with son's report*
PE	**General**: *alert x1 (name)*
	Skin: *rash on left side of torso (raised, erythema bullous − weeping − follows dermatome*
	Lungs: *CTA*
	Cardiac: *Normal rate and rhythm*
	Neuro: *some left sided weakness noted in upper and lower*
DIFF	*TIA, CVA, acute renal failure, sepsis, UTI*
Provider	*Discussed admission as inpatient with ER physician; spoke with neurologist and nephrology*
A/P	1. *Altered mental status: CT normal will obtain MRI of head and consult neurology*
	2. *Acute renal failure: suspect acyclovir to be the cause − reviewed labs done in ER − repeat BMP daily − give IV fluids − consult nephrology; stop acyclovir*
	3. *Sepsis: lactic acid is normal; will follow blood cultures, repeat CBC and serial lactic acid − hold antibiotics for now*
	4. *UTI: UA is normal* **ruled out**
Time	*55 minutes (review of records, examination of patient, coordination of care and documentation including orders)*

Table 6.8 Acute care initial or observation E/M codes

E/M code	History/Exam	MDM	Time
99221	Clinician required to perform and document medically appropriate history and examination	Straightforward or low	Or 40 minutes
99222		Moderate	Or 55 minutes
99223		High	Or 75 minutes

MDM = 99223 High

Time = 99222 Moderate

Table 6.9 Medical decision-making tool

MDM (2 out of 3 MDM)	Number of problems	Complexity of data reviewed	Risk of complications and or morbidity
Straightforward 99202 99212 99221 99231 99234	1 self-limited or minor problem	Minimal or NONE	Minimal risk of morbidity from additional diagnostic testing or treatment
Low complexity 99203 99213 99221 99231 99234	2 or more self-limited or minor problems *or* 1 stable, chronic illness *or* 1 acute uncomplicated illness or injury *or* 1 stable, acute illness *or* 1 acute, uncomplicated illness or injury requiring hospital inpatient or observation level of care	(Must meet 1 of 2 requirements) **Category 1: Tests and documents** Any combination of 2 from the following • Review of prior external note(s) from each unique source • Review of the result(s) of each unique test • Ordering of each unique test *or* **Category 2: Assessment requiring an independent historian(s)**	Low risk of morbidity from additional diagnostic testing or treatment

(Continued)

Table 6.9 (Continued)

MDM (2 out of 3 MDM)	Number of problems	Complexity of data reviewed	Risk of complications and or morbidity
Moderate	1 or more chronic illnesses with exacerbation, progression, or side effects of treatment	*(Must meet requirements of 1 out of 3)*	*Moderate risk of morbidity from additional diagnostic testing or treatment*
99204		**Category 1: Tests, documents, historian**	
99214		*Any combination of 3 from the following*	Examples only:
99222		• *Review of prior external note(s) from each unique source*	
99232	*or*	• *Review of the results (s) of each unique test*	• *Prescription drug management*
99235	2 or more stable chronic illnesses	• *Ordering of each unique test*	• *Decision regarding minor surgery with identified patient or procedure risk factors*
		• *Assessment requiring an independent historian(s)*	
	or	*or*	• *Decision regarding elective major surgery without identified patient or procedure risk factors*
	1 undiagnosed new problem with uncertain prognosis	**Category 2: Independent interpretation of tests**	
		• *Independent interpretation of a test performed by another physician/other qualified healthcare professional (not separately reported)*	• *Diagnosis or treatment significantly limited by social determinants of health*
	or	*or*	
	1 acute illness with systemic symptoms	**Category 3: Discussion of management or test interpretation**	
	or	• *Discussion of management or test interpretation with external/physician/ other qualified healthcare professional/appropriate source (not separately reported)*	
	1 acute, complicated injury		

High complexity

99205
99215
99223
99233
99236

1 or more chronic illnesses with severe exacerbation, progression, or side effects of treatment

or

1 acute or chronic illness or injury that poses a threat to life or bodily function

or

Multiple morbidities requiring intensive management (Initial Nursing Facility only)

(Must meet 2 out of 3 requirements)

Category 1: Tests, documents, historian

Any combination of 3 from the following Review of prior external note(s) from each unique source

- *Review of the result(s) of each unique test*
- *Ordering of each unique test*
- *Assessment requiring an independent historian(s)*

or

Category 2: Independent interpretation of tests

- *Independent interpretation of a test performed by another physician/other qualified healthcare professional (not separately reported)*

or

Category 3: Discussion of management or test interpretation

- *Discussion of management or test interpretation with external/physician/ other qualified healthcare professional/appropriate source (not separately reported)*

High risk of morbidity from additional diagnostic testing or treatment
Examples only:

- *Drug therapy requiring intensive monitoring for toxicity*
- *Decision for elective major surgery with identified patient or procedure risk factors*
- *Decision for emergency major surgery*
- *Decision regarding hospitalization*
- *Decision for DNR or to de-escalate care because of poor prognosis*
- *Parenteral controlled substances*

Table 6.10 Acute care (progress note) Subsequent hospital inpatient and observation services

CC	*Altered mental status*
HPI	*76-year-old female who lives alone in independent living, found by son confused in the bathroom covered with feces. States he and his mother went out to lunch earlier that day and she was fine. States she has recently been diagnosed with shingles and was started on some new medication, but he does not know the name of it. He is unaware of any previous kidney failure.*
Interval change	*Doing better today, more alert, knows she is in a hospital. Reviewed labs and noted improvement from 2.50 to 1.75 after fluids*
PE	**General:** *alert x2–3 (name, place, knows son)* **Skin**: *rash on left side of torso (raised, erythema bullous – weeping – follows dermatome* **Lungs**: *CTA* **Cardiac**: *Normal rate and rhythm* **Neuro**: *some left sided weakness noted in upper and lower* **BMP** *(creatinine 2.50 yesterday and today was 1.75)* *Potassium normal at 4.5*
Provider	*Discussed with nephrology – acute renal failure improving with fluids*
A/P	*1. Altered mental status – appears to have ruled out a CVA/ TIA – MRI is normal – improving with IV fluids* *2. Acute renal failure – resolving suspect acyclovir to be the cause – continue IV fluids and monitoring renal labs – nephrology is following* *3. Sepsis – ruled out* *4. UTI – ruled out*
Time	*35 minutes (review of records, examination of patient, coordination of care and documentation including orders)*

Table 6.11 Subsequent observation and inpatient E/M codes

E/M code	History/Exam	MDM	Time
99231	*Clinician required to perform and document medically appropriate history and examination*	*Straightforward or Low*	*Or 25 minutes*
99232		*Moderate*	*Or 35 minutes*
99233		*High*	*Or 50 minutes*

MDM = 99232 Moderate

Time = 99232 Moderate

Table 6.12 Medical decision-making tool

MDM (2 out of 3 MDM)	Number of problems	Complexity of data reviewed	Risk of complications and or morbidity
Straight forward 99202 99212 99221 99231 99234	1 self-limited or minor problem	Minimal or NONE	Minimal risk of morbidity from additional diagnostic testing or treatment
Low complexity 99203 99213 99221 99231 99234	2 or more self-limited or minor problems **or** 1 stable, chronic illness **or** 1 acute uncomplicated illness or injury **or** 1 stable, acute illness **or** 1 acute, uncomplicated illness or injury requiring hospital inpatient or observation level of care	(Must meet 1 of 2 requirements) **Category 1: Tests and documents** Any combination of 2 from the following • Review of prior external note(s) from each unique source • Review of the result(s) of each unique test • Ordering of each unique test **or** **Category 2: Assessment requiring an independent historian(s)**	Low risk of morbidity from additional diagnostic testing or treatment

Moderate	1 or more chronic illnesses with exacerbation, progression, or side effects of treatment	(Must meet requirements of 1 out of 3)	Moderate risk of morbidity from additional diagnostic testing or treatment
99204		**Category 1: Tests, documents, historian**	Examples only:
99214	**or**	Any combination of 3 from the following	
99222	2 or more stable chronic illnesses	• Review of prior external note(s) from each unique source	• Prescription drug management
99232		• Review of the result(s) of each unique test	• Decision regarding minor surgery
99235	**or**	• Ordering of each unique test	with identified patient or procedure risk factors
	1 undiagnosed new problem with uncertain prognosis	• Assessment requiring an independent historian(s)	• Decision regarding elective major surgery without identified patient or procedure risk factors
	or	**or**	• Diagnosis or treatment significantly limited by social determinants of health
	1 acute illness with systemic symptoms	**Category 2: Independent interpretation of tests**	
		• Independent interpretation of a test performed by another physician/other qualified healthcare professional not separately reported).	
	or	**or**	
	1 acute, complicated injury	**Category 3: Discussion of management or test interpretation**	
		• Discussion of management or test interpretation with external/physician/other qualified healthcare professional/appropriate source (not separately reported)	

(Continued)

Table 6.12 (Continued)

MDM (2 out of 3 MDM)	Number of problems	Complexity of data reviewed	Risk of complications and or morbidity
High complexity 99205 99215 99223 99233 99236	1 or more chronic illnesses with severe exacerbation, progression, or side effects of treatment **or** 1 acute or chronic illness or injury that poses a threat to life or bodily function **or** Multiple morbidities requiring intensive management (Initial Nursing Facility only)	*(Must meet 2 out of 3 requirements)* **Category 1: Tests, documents, historian** *Any combination of 3 from the following* • *Review of prior external note(s) from each unique source* • *Review of the result(s) of each unique test* • *Ordering of each unique test* • *Assessment requiring an independent historian(s)* **or** **Category 2: Independent interpretation of tests** • *Independent interpretation of a test performed by another physician/other qualified healthcare professional (not separately reported)* **or** **Category 3: Discussion of management or test interpretation** • *Discussion of management or test interpretation with external/physician/other qualified healthcare professional/appropriate source (not separately reported)*	High risk of morbidity from additional diagnostic testing or treatment Examples only: • *Drug therapy requiring intensive monitoring for toxicity* • *Decision for elective major surgery with identified patient or procedure risk factors* • *Decision for emergency major surgery* • *Decision regarding hospitalization* • *Decision for DNR or to de-escalate care because of poor prognosis* • *Parenteral controlled substances*

Table 6.13 Admit/discharge same day acute care

CC	**Chest pain**
HPI	*36 yo female admitted with exertional chest pain x 1 day. States it feels sharp. Complains of recent upper respiratory infection, also recently received COVID 19 vaccine and is worried about heart complications*
PFSH	*HTN – controlled on meds* *Father – died of heart attack at age 60* *Smokes 1 ppd x 20 years*
ROS	*General – no c/o fever* *Resp – c/o dry cough* *Cardiac – c/o sharp chest pain when she moves around*
PE	*General – well appearing* *Respiratory – CTA bilaterally* *Cardiac – Normal rate rhythm, no murmurs, pleural friction rub noted on LLL, no edema* *VS normal* *EKG shows NSR* *Cardiac troponins x3 with insignificant delta* *Stress test neg for ischemia* *Echo does not show pericardial effusion* *CXR – normal with no signs of infiltrate*
DIFF	*Rule out myocardial infarction, CAP, pericarditis (related to Covid 19 immunization)*
Provider	*Discussed with ED physician, decision to admit for stress test/echo and completion of cardiac enzymes; discussion with cardiology on results of echo*
Admission dx	**Rule out MI, acute coronary syndrome, pneumonia, pericarditis, pleural effusion, Pleuritic chest pain**

(Continued)

Table 6.13 (Continued)

CC	**Chest pain**
Discharge dx	*Pleuritic chest pain related to recent URI − given Toradol 30mg IM with relief/script for Naprosyn given*
	MI ruled out − EKG no changes with neg stress test
	Pneumonia ruled out − normal CXR
	Pleural effusion ruled out − normal echo with no signs of pericardial effusion
	Pericarditis ruled out − normal EKG
Dispo	*Home*
Code status	*Full*
Condition	*Good*
Discharge instructions	*Take Naprosyn 500mg BID for 7 days f/u with PCP in 1 week*
Time	*40 minutes*

Table 6.14 Admit/DC Same day: Observation E/M and inpatient service codes

E/M code	History/Exam	MDM	Time
99234-	*Clinician required to perform and document medically appropriate history and examination*	*Straightforward or Low*	*Or 40 minutes*
99235-		*Moderate*	*Or 70 minutes*
99236-		*High*	*Or 85 minutes*

MDM = 99236 High

Time = 99234 Straightforward or low

MDM (2 out of 3 MDM)	Number of problems	Complexity of data reviewed	Risk of complications and or morbidity
Straight forward 99202 99212 99221 99231 99234	1 self-limited or minor problem	Minimal or NONE	Minimal risk of morbidity from additional diagnostic testing or treatment
Low complexity 99203 99213 99221 99231 99234	2 or more self-limited or minor problems **or** 1 stable, chronic illness **or** 1 acute uncomplicated illness or injury **or** 1 stable, acute illness **or** 1 acute, uncomplicated illness or injury requiring hospital inpatient or observation level of care	(Must meet 1 of 2 requirements) **Category 1: Tests and documents** Any combination of 2 from the following • Review of prior external note(s) from each unique source • Review of the result(s) of each unique test • Ordering of each unique test **or** **Category 2: Assessment requiring an independent historian(s)**	Low risk of morbidity from additional diagnostic testing or treatment

(Continued)

Table 6.15 (Continued)

MDM (2 out of 3 MDM)	Number of problems	Complexity of data reviewed	Risk of complications and or morbidity
Moderate 99204 99214 99222 99232 99235	1 or more chronic illnesses with exacerbation, progression, or side effects of treatment or 2 or more stable chronic illnesses or 1 undiagnosed new problem with uncertain prognosis or 1 acute illness with systemic symptoms or 1 acute, complicated injury	(Must meet 1 out of 3 requirements) **Category 1: Tests, documents, historian** Any combination of 3 from the following • Review of prior external note(s) from each unique source • Review of the results (s) of each unique test • Ordering of each unique test • Assessment requiring an independent historian(s) or **Category 2: Independent interpretation of tests** • Independent interpretation of a test performed by another physician/other qualified healthcare professional (not separately reported). or **Category 3: Discuss of management or test interpretation.** • Discussion of management or test interpretation with external/physician/other qualified healthcare professional/appropriate source (not separately reported)	Moderate risk of morbidity from additional diagnostic testing or treatment Examples only: • Prescription drug management • Decision regarding minor surgery with identified patient or procedure risk factors • Decision regarding elective major surgery without identified patient or procedure risk factors • Diagnosis or treatment significantly limited by social determinants of health

High complexity

99205
99215
99223
99233
99236

1 or more chronic illnesses with severe exacerbation, progression, or side effects of treatment

or

1 acute or chronic illness or injury that poses a threat to life or bodily function

or

Multiple morbidities requiring intensive management (Initial Nursing Facility only)

(Must meet 2 out of 3 requirements)

Category 1: Tests, documents, historian

Any combination of 3 from the following

- *Review of prior external note(s) from each unique source*
- *Review of the result(s) of each unique test*
- *Ordering of each unique test*
- *Assessment requiring an independent historian(s)*

or

Category 2: Independent interpretation of tests

- *Independent interpretation of a test performed by another physician/other qualified healthcare professional (not separately reported)*

or

Category 3: Discussion of management or test interpretation

- *Discussion of management or test interpretation with external/physician/ other qualified healthcare professional/ appropriate source (not separately reported)*

High risk of morbidity from additional diagnostic testing or treatment

Examples only:

- *Drug therapy requiring intensive monitoring for toxicity*
- *Decision for elective major surgery with identified patient or procedure risk factors*
- *Decision for emergency major surgery*
- *Decision regarding hospitalization*
- *Decision for DNR or to de-escalate care because of poor prognosis*
- *Parenteral controlled substances*

Table 6.16 Hospital discharge day management E/M code

E/M code	Face-to-face encounter	Time
99238	Clinician required to perform and document medically appropriate history and examination	≤ 30 minutes
99239		≥ 30 minutes

Table 6.17 Hospital discharge 99238 example

Day of admission	10/5/2022
Day of discharge	10/7/2022
Discharge diagnosis	Cellulitis RLE
Brief physical exam	Alert and oriented x3 RLE with minimal redness, warmth, no pain Resp – CTA Cardiac – RRR
Hospital course	76-year-old male with history of DM type 2 came in with c/o RLE redness warmth and pain. Treated with IV Vancomycin with improvement in symptoms, discharged on Doxycycline.
Discharge meds	Doxycycline 100mg BID for 7 days
Additional tests	No further tests needed
Follow up	f/u with primary care doctor in 7 days
Dispo	Home
Condition	Good
Time	Total time spent in review of record, physical exam, coordination of care with care givers and preparation of discharge paperwork is 30 minutes

Time ≤ 30 minutes = 99238

Table 6.18 Hospital discharge day management E/M code

E/M code	Face-to-face encounter	Time
99238	*Clinician required to perform and document medically appropriate history and examination*	*≤ 30 minutes*
99239		*≥ 30 minutes*

Table 6.19 Hospital discharge 99239 example

Day of admission	*10/5/2022*
Day of discharge	*10/7/2022*
Discharge diagnosis	*Cellulitis RLE*
Brief physical exam	*Alert and oriented x3* *RLE with minimal redness, warmth, no pain* *Resp – CTA* *Cardiac – RRR*
Hospital course	*76-year-old male with history of DM type 2 came in with c/o RLE redness warmth and pain. Treated with IV Vancomycin with improvement in symptoms, discharged on Doxycycline.*
Discharge meds	*Doxycycline 100mg BID for 7 days*
Additional tests	*No further tests needed*
Follow up	*f/u with primary care doctor in 7 days*
Dispo	*Home*
Condition	*Good*
Time	*Total time spent in review of record, physical exam, coordination of care with care givers and preparation of discharge paperwork is __ 35_minutes*

Time > 30 minutes = 99239

EMERGENCY ROOM

- No distinction between new or established patient.
- IF critical care services provided in the ER follow 99291, 99292.
- Critical care and ER services may both be reported on the same day IF after completion of the ER services critical care services are needed.
- For observation or inpatient services utilize codes 99221, 99222, or 99223 for the initial encounter and 99231, 99232, 99233, 99238, or 99239 for subsequent or discharge encounters.
- For same day inpatient or observation care services utilize 99234, 99235, 99236.
- For services provide in the ED for convenience of a physician or other qualified healthcare professional, use the office or other outpatient services codes (99202–99215)
- TIME is NOT a factor in the ER setting.

Table 6.20 Emergency room sample note

CC	*Cold symptoms*
HPI	*24 yo female came with c/o nasal congestion and pain for past 2 weeks with a scratchy throat and fever x2 days. She has been exposed to influenza at school and COVID 19*
PFSH	*No significant PMH*
ROS	*General: c/o fever* *HEENT: c/o sinus pressure and drainage that is yellow and thick last 2 days, c/o scratchy throat* *Resp: c/o dry cough* *GI: no c/o nausea or vomiting*
PE	*General: well appearing* *HEENT: maxillary pressure with thick yellow drainage in nares, throat with erythema and exudate*
DIFF	*Bacterial sinus infection, Influenza A, COVID 19*
Provider	*NA*

(Continued)

Table 6.20 (Continued)

Testing	*Strep rapid – neg* *Covid rapid – neg* *Flu A/B – positive for A*
Dx	*Influenza A – Tamiflu prescribed and supportive care* *Flonase/Tessalon pearls*
Discharge instructions	*Influenza A information given with supportive means, complete all medications*
Time	*30 minutes*

Table 6.21 Emergency room E/M code

E/M code	History/Exam	MDM
99281	*Clinician required to perform and document medically appropriate history and examination*	*N/A*
99282		*Straightforward*
99283		*Low*
99284		*Moderate*
99285		*High*

MDM=99283 Low

NO TIME component

Table 6.22 Medical decision-making tool

MDM (2 out of 3 MDM)	Number of problems	Complexity of data reviewed	Risk of complications and or morbidity
Straightforward 99202 99212 99221 99231 99234	1 self-limited or minor problem	Minimal or NONE	Minimal risk of morbidity from additional diagnostic testing or treatment
Low complexity 99203 99213 99221 99231 99234	2 or more self-limited or minor problems or 1 stable, chronic illness or 1 acute uncomplicated illness or injury or 1 stable, acute illness or 1 acute, uncomplicated illness or injury requiring hospital inpatient or observation level of care	(Must meet 1 of 2 requirements) **Category 1: Tests and documents** Any combination of 2 from the following • Review of prior external note(s) from each unique source • Review of the result(s) of each unique test • Ordering of each unique test or **Category 2: Assessment requiring an independent historian(s)**	Low risk of morbidity from additional diagnostic testing or treatment

Moderate		(Must meet requirements of 1 out of 3)	Moderate risk of morbidity from additional diagnostic testing or treatment
99204 99214 99222 99232 99235	1 or more chronic illnesses with exacerbation, progression, or side effects of treatment **or** 2 or more stable chronic illnesses **or** 1 undiagnosed new problem with uncertain prognosis **or** 1 acute illness with systemic symptoms **or** 1 acute, complicated injury	**Category 1: Tests, documents, historian** Any combination of 3 from the following • Review of prior external note(s) from each unique source • Review of the result(s) of each unique test • Ordering of each unique test • Assessment requiring an independent historian(s) **or** **Category 2: Independent interpretation of tests** • Independent interpretation of a test performed by another physician/other qualified healthcare professional (not separately reported) **or** **Category 3: Discussion of management or test interpretation** • Discussion of management or test interpretation with external/physician/other qualified healthcare professional/appropriate source (not separately reported)	Examples only: • Prescription drug management • Decision regarding minor surgery with identified patient or procedure risk factors • Decision regarding elective major surgery without identified patient or procedure risk factors • Diagnosis or treatment significantly limited by social determinants of health

(Continued)

Table 6.22 (Continued)

MDM (2 out of 3 MDM)	Number of problems	Complexity of data reviewed	Risk of complications and or morbidity
High complexity 99205 99215 99223 99233 99236	*1 or more chronic illnesses with severe exacerbation, progression, or side effects of treatment,* **or** *1 acute or chronic illness or injury that poses a threat to life or bodily function* **or** *Multiple morbidities requiring intensive management (Initial Nursing Facility only)*	*(Must meet 2 out of 3 requirements of)* **Category 1: Tests, documents, historian** *Any combination of 3 from the following* • *Review of prior external note(s) from each unique source* • *Review of the result(s) of each unique test* • *Ordering of each unique test* • *Assessment requiring an independent historian(s)* **or** **Category 2: Independent interpretation of tests** • *Independent interpretation of a test performed by another physician/other qualified healthcare professional (not separately reported)* **or** **Category 3: Discussion of management or test interpretation** • *Discussion of management or test interpretation with external/physician/ other qualified healthcare professional/ appropriate source (not separately reported)*	*High risk of morbidity from additional diagnostic testing or treatment* Examples only: • *Drug therapy requiring intensive monitoring for toxicity* • *Decision for elective major surgery with identified patient or procedure risk factors* • *Decision for emergency major surgery* • *Decision regarding hospitalization* • *Decision for DNR or to de-escalate care because of poor prognosis* • *Parenteral controlled substances*

Table 6.23 Consultations – office or other outpatient consults

CC	Hyperparathyroidism
HPI	56-year-old female found to have elevated calcium of 10.6 on routine labs. PTH was checked and found to be elevated. Pt referred for suspected hyperparathyroidism.
PFSH	PMH – HTN
ROS	General: no weight loss or gain Resp: no c/o SOB/wheezing Cardiac: no c/o palpitations/DOE Endocrine: denies feeling cold/hot/constipation/diarrhea/dry or oily skin Psych: denies depression or anxiety
PE	VS 138/76 HR: 88 R: 16 Weight: 155 Height: 5' 6"
A/P	Hyperparathyroidism – will obtain thyroid ultrasound; check BMP – discussed surgery to remove enlarged parathyroid gland with risks and benefits discussed
Time	55 minutes spent in review of previous records, examination of patient, counseling regarding necessary surgery, and ordering further testing.

Table 6.24 Office or other outpatient consults E/M codes

E/M code	History/Exam	MDM	Time
99242	Clinician required to perform and document medically appropriate history and examination	Straightforward	Or 20 minutes
99243		Low complexity	Or 30 minutes
99244		Mod complexity	Or 40 minutes
99245		High complexity	Or 55 minutes

MDM = 99244 Moderate

TIME = 99245 High

Table 6.25 Medical decision-making tool

MDM (2 out of 3 MDM)	Number of problems	Complexity of data reviewed	Risk of complications and or morbidity
Straight forward 99202 99212 99221 99231 99234	1 self-limited or minor problem	Minimal or NONE	Minimal risk of morbidity from additional diagnostic testing or treatment
Low complexity 99203 99213 99221 99231 99234	2 or more self-limited or minor problems, *or* 1 stable, chronic illness, *or* 1 acute uncomplicated illness or injury *or* 1 stable, acute illness *or* 1 acute, uncomplicated illness or injury requiring hospital inpatient or observation level of care	*(Must meet 1 of 2 requirements)* **Category 1: Tests and documents** Any combination of 2 from the following Review of prior external note(s) from each unique source Review of the result(s) of each unique test Ordering of each unique test *or* **Category 2: Assessment requiring an independent historian(s)**	Low risk of morbidity from additional diagnostic testing or treatment

Moderate		(Must meet 1 out of 3 requirements of)	Moderate risk of morbidity from additional diagnostic testing or treatment
99204	1 or more chronic illnesses with exacerbation, progression, or side effects of treatment	**Category 1: Tests, documents, historian**	Examples only:
99214		Any combination of 3 from the following	
99222	**or**	• Review of prior external note(s) from each unique source	• Prescription drug management
99232	2 or more stable chronic illnesses	• Review of the result(s) of each unique test	• Decision regarding minor surgery with identified patient or procedure risk factors
99235		• Ordering of each unique test	
	or	• Assessment requiring an independent historian(s)	• Decision regarding elective major surgery without identified patient or procedure risk factors
	1 undiagnosed new problem with uncertain prognosis	**or**	
		Category 2: Independent interpretation of tests	• Diagnosis or treatment significantly limited by social determinants of health
	or	• Independent interpretation of a test peformed by another physician/other qualified healthcare professional (not separately reported)	
	1 acute illness with systemic symptoms	**or**	
	or	**Category 3: Discussion of management or test interpretation**	
	1 acute, complicated injury	• Discussion of mangement or test interpretation with external/physician/other qualified healthcare professional/appropriate source (not separately reported)	

(Continued)

Table 6.25 (Continued)

MDM (2 out of 3 MDM)	Number of problems	Complexity of data reviewed	Risk of complications and or morbidity
High complexity 99205 99215 99223 99233 99236	1 or more chronic illnesses with severe exacerbation, progression, or side effects of treatment or 1 acute or chronic illness or injury that poses a threat to life or bodily function or Multiple morbidities requiring intensive management (Initial Nursing Facility only)	*(Must meet 2 out of 3 requirements)* **Category 1: Tests, documents, historian** *Any combination of 3 from the following* • *Review of prior external note(s) from each unique source* • *Review of the result(s) of each unique test* • *Ordering of each unique test* • *Assessment requiring an independent historian(s)* **or** **Category 2: Independent interpretation of tests** • *Independent interpretation of a test performed by another physician/other qualified healthcare professional (not separately reported)* **or** **Category 3: Discussion of management or test interpretation** • *Discussion of management or test interpretation with external/physician/other qualified healthcare professional/appropriate source (not separately reported)*	*High risk of morbidity from additional diagnostic testing or treatment* Examples only: • *Drug therapy requiring intensive monitoring for toxicity* • *Decision for elective major surgery with identified patient or procedure risk factors* • *Decision for emergency major surgery* • *Decision regarding hospitalization* • *Decision for DNR or to de-escalate care because of poor prognosis* • *Parenteral controlled substances*

Table 6.26 Example of inpatient consultation

CC	*Hyperparathyroidism*
HPI	*56-year-old female found to have elevated calcium of 10.6 on routine labs. PTH was checked and found to be elevated. Pt referred for suspected hyperparathyroidism.*
PFSH	*PMH – HTN*
ROS	*General: no weight loss or gain* *Resp: no c/o SOB/wheezing* *Cardiac: no c/o palpitations/DOE* *Endocrine: denies feeling cold/hot/constipation/diarrhea/dry or oily skin* *Psych- denies depression or anxiety*
PE	*VS 138/76 HR: 88 R: 16 Weight: 155 Height: 5' 6"*
A/P	*Hyperparathyroidism – will obtain thyroid ultrasound; check BMP – discussed surgery to remove enlarged parathyroid gland with risks and benefits discussed*
Time	*55 minutes spent in review of previous records, examination of patient, counseling regarding necessary surgery, and ordering further testing.*

Table 6.27 Inpatient consultation E/M codes

E/M code	History/Exam	MDM	Time
99252	*Clinician required to perform and document medically appropriate history and examination*	*Straight forward*	*Or 35 minutes*
99253		*Low Complexity*	*Or 45 minutes*
99254		*Mod Complexity*	*Or 60 minutes*
99255		*High Complexity*	*Or 80 minutes*

MDM = 99254 Moderate

Time = 99253 Low

Table 6.28 Medical decision-making tool

MDM (2 out of 3 MDM)	Number of problems	Complexity of data reviewed	Risk of complications and or morbidity
Straight forward 99202 99212 99221 99231 99234	1 self-limited or minor problem	Minimal or NONE	Minimal risk of morbidity from additional diagnostic testing or treatment
Low complexity 99203 99213 99221 99231 99234	2 or more self-limited or minor problems or 1 stable, chronic illness or 1 acute uncomplicated illness or injury or 1 stable, acute illness or 1 acute, uncomplicated illness or injury requiring hospital inpatient or observation level of care	(Must meet 1 of 2 requirements) **Category 1: Tests and documents** Any combination of 2 from the following • Review of prior external note(s) from each unique source • Review of the result(s) of each unique test • Ordering of each unique test or **Category 2: Assessment requiring an independent historian(s)**	Low risk of morbidity from additional diagnostic testing or treatment

Moderate			
99204			
99214			
99222			
99232			
99235			

Moderate

1 or more chronic illnesses with exacerbation, progression, or side effects of treatment

or

2 or more stable chronic illnesses

or

1 undiagnosed new problem with uncertain prognosis

or

1 acute illness with systemic symptoms

or

1 acute, complicated injury

(Must meet 1 out of 3 requirements)

Category 1: Tests, documents, historian

Any combination of 3 from the following

- Review of prior external note(s) from each unique source
- Review of the result(s) of each unique test
- Ordering of each unique test
- Assessment requiring an independent historian(s)

or

Category 2: Independent interpretation of tests

- Independent interpretation of a test performed by another physician/other qualified healthcare professional (not separately reported).

or

Category 3: Discussion of management or test interpretation

- Discussion of management or test interpretation with external/physician/other qualified healthcare professional/appropriate source (not separately reported)

Moderate risk of morbidity from additional diagnostic testing or treatment

Examples only:

- Prescription drug management
- Decision regarding minor surgery with identified patient or procedure risk factors
- Decision regarding elective major surgery without identified patient or procedure risk factors
- Diagnosis or treatment significantly limited by social determinants of health

(Continued)

Table 6.28 (Continued)

MDM (2 out of 3 MDM)	Number of problems	Complexity of data reviewed	Risk of complications and or morbidity
High complexity 99205 99215 99223 99233 99236	*1 or more chronic illnesses with severe exacerbation, progression, or side effects of treatment* **or** *1 acute or chronic illness or injury that poses a threat to life or bodily function* **or** *Multiple morbidities requiring intensive management (Initial Nursing Facility only)*	*(Must meet 2 out of 3 requirements)* **Category 1: Tests, documents, historian** *Any combination of 3 from the following* • *Review of prior external note(s) from each unique source* • *Review of the result(s) of each unique test* • *Ordering of each unique test* • *Assessment requiring an independent historian(s)* **or** **Category 2: Independent interpretation of tests** • *Independent interpretation of a test performed by another physician/other qualified healthcare professional (not separately reported).* **or** **Category 3: Discussion of management or test interpretation** • *Discussion of management or test interpretation with external/physician/other qualified healthcare professional/appropriate source (not separately reported)*	*High risk of morbidity from additional diagnostic testing or treatment* Examples only: • *Drug therapy requiring intensive monitoring for toxicity* • *Decision for elective major surgery with identified patient or procedure risk factors* • *Decision for emergency major surgery* • *Decision regarding hospitalization* • *Decision for DNR or to de-escalate care because of poor prognosis* • *Parenteral controlled substances*

Table 6.29 Skilled Nursing Facility Services: Initial visit

CC	*S/P Right hip repair*
HPI	*67-year-old female out walking her dog fell and felt pop in right hip and was unable to stand. Taken to ER where she was found to have a right hip fracture which was repaired with intertrochanter hip nailing.*
PFSH	*PMH – includes, HTN, CAD s/p stent, HLD, and DM type 2*
ROS	*General: no complaints of recent weight loss or gain* *Respiratory: no c/o cough or shortness of breath* *Cardiac: no c/o chest pain or DOE* *Muscular skeletal: c/o right leg feeling heavy, with pain when she moves it* *Psych: no c/o depression or anxiety*
PE	*Vital signs: 167/88 84 16 98.6* *General: alert, well appearing female in no distress* *Respiratory: lungs CTA* *Cardiac: RRR with no murmurs or clicks* *Muscular skeletal: Right hip dressing clean, dry, and intact with some right leg swelling, calf nontender, neg Homans sign* *Psych: answers questions appropriately with good insight*
A/P	*ORIF right HIP s/p intertrochanter fracture – PT/OT/wound care/monitor for signs of infection* *Acute blood loss anemia – CBC every 3 days transfuse if hemoglobin < 7-* *HTN – continue home meds* *CAD s/p Stent – on Plavix and ASA, ACE, BB* *HLD – continue statin* *DM type 2 – monitor blood sugars/sliding scale insulin as needed* *DVT prophylaxis – on ASA 325 mg BID – continue PPI to protect stomach*
Time	*Total time spent 50 minutes in review of hospital records, examination of patient, finalization of admission orders to include medication reconciliation, and ordering of lab work.*

Table 6.30 E/M codes for Initial Nursing Facility Services

E/M code	History/Exam	MDM	Time
99304	*Clinician required to perform and document medically appropriate history and examination*	*Straight forward or low*	*Or 25 minutes*
99305		*Moderate*	*Or 35 minutes*
99306		High	*Or 45 minutes*

MDM = 99305 Moderate

TIME = 99306 High

Table 6.31 Medical decision-making tool

MDM (2 out of 3 MDM)	Number of problems	Complexity of data reviewed	Risk of complications and or morbidity
Straightforward 99202 99212 99221 99231 99234	*1 self-limited or minor problem*	*Minimal or NONE*	*Minimal risk of morbidity from additional diagnostic testing or treatment*
Low complexity 99203 99213 99221 99231 99234	*2 or more self-limited or minor problems* or *1 stable, chronic illness,* or *1 acute uncomplicated illness or injury* or *1 stable, acute illness* or *1 acute, uncomplicated illness or injury requiring hospital inpatient or observation level of care*	*(Must meet 1 of 2 requirements)* **Category 1: Tests and documents** *Any combination of 2 from the following* • *Review of prior external note(s) from each unique source* • *Review of the result(s) of each unique test* • *Ordering of each unique test* **OR** **Category 2: Assessment requiring an independent historian(s)**	*Low risk of morbidity from additional diagnostic testing or treatment*

(Continued)

Table 6.31 (Continued)

MDM (2 out of 3 MDM)	Number of problems	Complexity of data reviewed	Risk of complications and or morbidity
Moderate 99204 99214 99222 99232 99235	1 or more chronic illnesses with exacerbation, progression, or side effects of treatment *or* 2 or more stable chronic illnesses *or* 1 undiagnosed new problem with uncertain prognosis *or* 1 acute illness with systemic symptoms *or* 1 acute, complicated injury	*(Must meet 1 out of 3 requirements)* **Category 1: Tests, documents, historian** *Any combination of 3 from the following* • *Review of prior external note(s) from each unique source* • *Review of the result(s) of each unique test* • *Ordering of each unique test* • *Assessment requiring an independent historian(s)* *or* **Category 2: Independent interpretation of tests** • *Independent interpretation of a test performed by another physician/other qualified healthcare professional not separately reported).* *or* **Category 3: Discussion of management or test interpretation** • *Discussion of management or test interpretation with external/physician/ other qualified healthcare professional/appropriate source (not separately reported)*	*Moderate risk of morbidity from additional diagnostic testing or treatment* Examples only: • *Prescription drug-management* • *Decision regarding minor surgery with identified patient or procedure risk factors* • *Decision regarding elective major surgery without identified patient or procedure risk factors* • *Diagnosis or treatment significantly limited by social determinants of health*

| **High complexity**
99205
99215
99223
99233
99236 | 1 or more chronic illnesses with severe exacerbation, progression, or side effects of treatment

or

1 acute or chronic illness or injury that poses a threat to life or bodily function

or

Multiple morbidities requiring intensive management (Initial Nursing Facility only) | *(Must meet 2 out of 3 requirements)*
Category 1: Tests, documents, historian
Any combination of 3 from the following
• *Review of prior external note(s) from each unique source*
• *Review of the result(s) of each unique test*
• *Ordering of each unique test*
• *Assessment requiring an independent historian(s)*

or

Category 2: Independent interpretation of tests
• *Independent interpretation of a test performed by another physician/other qualified healthcare professional not separately reported).*

or

Category 3: Discussion of management or test interpretation
• *Discussion of management or test interpretation with external/physician/other qualified healthcare professional/appropriate source (not separately reported)* | *High risk of morbidity from additional diagnostic testing or treatment*
Examples only:

• *Drug therapy requiring intensive monitoring for toxicity*
• *Decision for elective major surgery with identified patient or procedure risk factors*
• *Decision for emergency major surgery*
• *Decision regarding hospitalization*
• *Decision for DNR or to de-escalate care because of poor prognosis*
• *Parenteral controlled substances* |

Table 6.32 Skilled Nursing Facility Services: Subsequent visit

CC	*Right hip repair*
HPI	*67-year-old female out walking her dog fell and felt pop in right hip and was unable to stand. Taken to ER where she was found to have a right hip fracture which was repaired with intertrochanter hip nailing.*
Interval development	*Pt doing well in therapy — review of labs indicates hemoglobin dropped from 8.6 to 6.5 — swelling to right leg has increased, pt is c/o being tired and BP has been low 90/60.*
PE	*VS 100/80 P 100 R 20* *General: pt appears fatigued* *Skin: pale in color* *HEENT: conjunctiva pale* *Resp: CTA* *Cardiac: RRR* *Extremities: RLE increased with swelling, neg Homans sign calf soft — incision line without signs of infection*
A/P	*ORIF right HIP s/p intertrochanter fracture — PT/OT/ wound care/monitor for signs of infection — swelling has increased will get ultrasound of RLE to check for bleeding* *Acute blood loss anemia — Transfuse 1-unit pRBCs-* *Hypotension — hold BP meds; start IV fluids NS at 100cc/ hour* *CAD s/p Stent — Hold ASA and Plavix for now* *DM type 2 — monitor blood sugars/sliding scale insulin as needed* *DVT prophylaxis — SCDs for now*
Provider	*Discussed with attending physician change in status — will hold PT/OT today and get ultrasound of RLE and hold anticoagulants — if ultrasound shows positive for subcutaneous bleeding will transfer to hospital.*
Time	*Total time spent in review of records, examination of patient, discussion with provider, documentation and ordering of tests, as well as updated family 45 minutes*

Table 6.33 Subsequent visit E/M codes for Nursing Facility Services

E/M code	History/Exam	MDM	Time
99307	Clinician required to perform and document medically appropriate history and examination	Straightforward	Or 10 minutes
99308		LOW	Or 15 minutes
99309		Moderate	Or 30 minutes
99310		HIGH	Or 45 minutes

MDM = 99310 High

TIME = 99310 High

Table 6.34 Medical decision-making tool

MDM (2 out of 3 MDM)	Number of problems	Complexity of data reviewed	Risk of complications and or morbidity
Straight forward 99202 99212 99221 99231 99234	*1 self-limited or minor problem*	*Minimal or NONE*	*Minimal risk of morbidity from additional diagnostic testing or treatment*
Low complexity 99203 99213 99221 99231 99234	*2 or more self-limited or minor problems* **or** *1 stable, chronic illness* **or** *1 acute uncomplicated illness or injury* **or** *1 stable, acute illness* **or** *1 acute, uncomplicated illness or injury requiring hospital inpatient or observation level of care*	*(Must meet 1 of 2 requirements)* **Category 1: Tests and documents** *Any combination of 2 from the following* • *Review of prior external note(s) from each unique source* • *Review of the result(s) of each unique test* • *Ordering of each unique test* **or** **Category 2: Assessment requiring an independent historian(s)**	*Low risk of morbidity from additional diagnostic testing or treatment*

Moderate

99204
99214
99222
99232
99235

1 or more chronic illnesses with exacerbation, progression, or side effects of treatment

or

2 or more stable chronic illnesses

or

1 undiagnosed new problem with uncertain prognosis

or

1 acute illness with systemic symptoms

or

1 acute, complicated injury

(Must meet requirements of 1 out of 3)

Category 1: Tests, documents, historian

Any combination of 3 from the following

- Review of prior external note(s) from each unique source
- Review of the result(s) of each unique test
- Ordering of each unique test
- Assessment requiring an independent historian(s)

or

Category 2: Independent interpretation of tests

- Independent interpretation of a test performed by another physician/other qualified healthcare professional not separately reported).

or

Category 3: Discussion of management or test interpretation

- Discussion of management or test interpretation with external/physician/ other qualified healthcare professional/appropriate source (not separately reported)

Moderate risk of morbidity from additional diagnostic testing or treatment

Examples only:

- Prescription drug management
- Decision regarding minor surgery with identified patient or procedure risk factors
- Decision regarding elective major surgery without identified patient or procedure risk factors
- Diagnosis or treatment significantly limited by social determinants of health

(Continued)

Table 6.34 (Continued)

MDM (2 out of 3 MDM)	Number of problems	Complexity of data reviewed	Risk of complications and or morbidity
High complexity 99205 99215 99223 99233 99236	1 or more chronic illnesses with severe exacerbation, progression, or side effects of treatment **or** 1 acute or chronic illness or injury that poses a threat to life or bodily function **or** Multiple morbidities requiring intensive management (Initial Nursing Facility only)	*(Must meet 2 out of 3 requirements of)* **Category 1: Tests, documents, historian** *Any combination of 3 from the following* • *Review of prior external note(s) from each unique source* • *Review of the result(s) of each unique test* • *Ordering of each unique test* • *Assessment requiring an independent historian(s)* **Category 2: Independent interpretation of tests** • *Independent interpretation of a test performed by another physician/other qualified healthcare professional not separately reported).* **or** **Category 3: Discussion of management or test interpretation** • *Discussion of management or test interpretation with external/physician/other qualified healthcare professional/appropriate source (not separately reported)*	High risk of morbidity from additional diagnostic testing or treatment Examples only: • *Drug therapy requiring intensive monitoring for toxicity* • *Decision for elective major surgery with identified patient or procedure risk factors* • *Decision for emergency major surgery* • *Decision regarding hospitalization* • *Decision for DNR or to de-escalate care because of poor prognosis* • *Parenteral controlled substances*

Table 6.35 Discharge Nursing Facility Services E/M billing code

E/M code	Face-to-face encounter	Time
99215 – Discharge	Face-to-face encounter with the patient, family and/or caregiver required. May be performed on a date prior to the date the patient leaves the facility	≤ 30 minutes
99216 – Discharge		≥ 30 minutes

Table 6.36 Example discharge nursing facility note 99215

Day of admission	9/26/2022
Day of discharge	10/5/2022
Discharge diagnosis	Right hip intertrochanter fracture with hip nailing
Brief physical exam	VS 120/80 p 88 r 16 t 98.6 Alert x3 Lungs – CTA Cardiac – RRR Extremities – Right hip with minimal swelling, no tenderness, incision line clean and dry, good pedal pulses, calf is soft with neg Homans sign CBC shows hemoglobin of 8.5 and stable
Course	Pt admitted for rehab from intertrochanter right hip nailing and did well with PT/OT. Noted to have a drop in hemoglobin requiring transfusion of 1unit pRBC. Right leg noted to increase in swelling, anticoagulants held (Plavix and ASA) until right leg ultrasound done. Right hip ultrasound did not show any active bleeding – discussed with cardiology need for Plavix and since it has been greater than 1 year since stent placed okay to hold Plavix, resumed ASA 325 mg BID and continued PPI for stomach protection. Pt discharge hemoglobin is 8.5 and has been stable. Pt stable for discharge to home.

(Continued)

Table 6.36 (Continued)

Discharge meds	Resume home meds
	Continue ASA 325mg BID for next 2 weeks
	Then resume Plavix 75mg daily and ASA 81mg daily
Additional tests	Repeat CBC in 1 week
Follow up	f/u with orthopedic surgeon in 1 week
Dispo	Home
Condition	Good
Time	Time spent in review of record, examination of patient, coordination of care and preparation of DC paperwork 25 minutes.

Table 6.37 Discharge Nursing Facility Services E/M billing code

E/M code	Face-to-face encounter	Time
99215-Discharge	Face to face encounter with the patient, family and/or caregiver required. May be performed on a date prior to the date the patient leaves the facility	≤ 30 minutes
99216-Discharge		≥30 minutes

Table 6.38 Example discharge nursing facility note 99216

Day of admission	9/26/2022
Day of discharge	10/5/2022
Discharge diagnosis	Right hip intertrochanter fracture with hip nailing
Brief physical exam	VS 120/80 p 88 r 16 t 98.6
	Alert x3
	Lungs – CTA
	Cardiac – RRR
	Extremities – Right hip with minimal swelling, no tenderness, incision line clean and dry, good pedal pulses, calf is soft with neg Homans sign

(Continued)

Table 6.38 (Continued)

	CBC shows hemoglobin of 8.5 and stable
Course	*Pt admitted for rehab from intertrochanter right hip nailing and did well with PT/OT. Noted to have a drop in hemoglobin requiring transfusion of 1 unit pRBC. Right leg noted to increase in swelling, anticoagulants held (Plavix and ASA) until right leg ultrasound done. Right hip ultrasound did not show any active bleeding – discussed with cardiology need for Plavix and since it has been greater than 1 year since stent placed okay to hold Plavix, resumed ASA 325 mg BID and continued PPI for stomach protection. Pt discharge hemoglobin is 8.5 and has been stable. Pt stable for discharge to home.*
Discharge meds	*Resume home meds* *Continue ASA 325mg BID for next 2 weeks* *Then resume Plavix 75mg daily and ASA 81 mg daily*
Additional tests	*Repeat CBC in 1 week*
Follow up	*f/u with orthopedic surgeon in 1 week*
Dispo	*Home*
Condition	*Good*
Time	*Time spent in review of record, examination of patient, coordination of care and preparation of DC paperwork 35 minutes.*

Table 6.39 Domiciliary, rest home, or custodial care services – new patient

CC	*Weakness*
HPI	*86-year-old female admitted to hospital because family states they could no longer take care of her. Pt has been admitted multiple times for falling, does not participate well with PT/OT and appetite is variable.*
PFSH	*PMH – includes h/o CVA with left sided weakness, HTN*
ROS	*General: pt reports feeling tired and has no appetite.* *Respiratory: pt denies SOB or cough* *Cardiac: pt denies heart racing or chest pain* *Muscular skeletal: pt reports frequent back pain which is chronic* *Psych: pt reports feeling depressed*
PE	*VS 142/86 p 88 r 16 t 98.6* *General: well developed female who appears her stated age* *Respiratory: CTA* *Cardiac: RRR with no murmurs or clicks* *Abdomen: large, soft, normal bowel sounds* *Neurological: generalized weakness* *Psych: flat affect*
A/P	*Hypertension: resume home meds* *h/o CVA: daily range of motion, encourage to be up – continue ASA and statin* *Polypharmacy: review medications and eliminate as many as possible* *Depression: PHQ-9 screens positive for depression after interview she meets criteria for Major Depressive Disorder will start on Zoloft 25mg daily*
TIME	*45 minutes spent in review of records, examination of patient, documentation and placing orders*

Table 6.40 Domiciliary, rest home, or custodial care services – new patient E/M codes

E/M code	History/Exam	MDM	Time
99341 – NEW	Clinician required to perform and document medically appropriate history and examination	Straightforward	Or 15 minutes
99342 – NEW		Low complexity	Or 30 minutes
99344 – NEW		Mod complexity	Or 60 minutes
99345 – NEW		High complexity	Or 75 minutes

MDM = 99344 Moderate

TIME = 99342 Moderate

Table 6.41 Medical decision-making tool

MDM (2 out of 3 MDM)	Number of problems	Complexity of data reviewed	Risk of complications and or morbidity
Straightforward 99202 99212 99221 99231 99234	1 self-limited or minor problem	Minimal or NONE	Minimal risk of morbidity from additional diagnostic testing or treatment
Low complexity 99203 99213 99221 99231 99234	2 or more self-limited or minor problems or 1 stable, chronic illness or 1 acute uncomplicated illness or injury or 1 stable, acute illness or 1 acute, uncomplicated illness or injury requiring hospital inpatient or observation level of care	(Must meet 1 of 2 requirements) **Category 1: Tests and documents** Any combination of 2 from the following • Review of prior external note(s) from each unique source • Review of the result(s) of each unique test • Ordering of each unique test or **Category 2: Assessment requiring an independent historian(s)**	Low risk of morbidity from additional diagnostic testing or treatment

| **Moderate**
99204
99214
99222
99232
99235 | 1 or more chronic illnesses with exacerbation, progression, or side effects of treatment

or

2 or more stable chronic illnesses

or

1 undiagnosed new problem with uncertain prognosis

or

1 acute illness with systemic symptoms

or

1 acute, complicated injury | (Must meet 1 out of 3 requirements)
Category 1: Tests, documents, historian
Any combination of 3 from the following
• Review of prior external note(s) from each unique source
• Review of the result(s) of each unique test
• Ordering of each unique test
• Assessment requiring an independent historian(s)
or
Category 2: Independent interpretation of tests
• Independent interpretation of a test performed by another physician/other qualified healthcare professional (not separately reported).
or
Category 3: Discussion of management or test interpretation
• Discussion of management or test interpretation with external/physician/ other qualified healthcare professional/appropriate source (not separately reported) | Moderate risk of morbidity from additional diagnostic testing or treatment
Examples only:

• Prescription drug management
• Decision regarding minor surgery with identified patient or procedure risk factors
• Decision regarding elective major surgery without identified patient or procedure risk factors
• Diagnosis or treatment significantly limited by social determinants of health |

(Continued)

Table 6.41 (Continued)

MDM (2 out of 3 MDM)	Number of problems	Complexity of data reviewed	Risk of complications and or morbidity
High complexity 99205 99215 99223 99233 99236	1 or more chronic illnesses with severe exacerbation, progression, or side effects of treatment or 1 acute or chronic illness or injury that poses a threat to life or bodily function or Multiple morbidities requiring intensive management (Initial Nursing Facility only)	*(Must meet 2 out of 3 requirements)* **Category 1: Tests, documents, historian** *Any combination of 3 from the following* • *Review of prior external note(s) from each unique source* • *Review of the result(s) of each unique test* • *Ordering of each unique test* • *Assessment requiring an independent historian(s)* **or** **Category 2: Independent interpretation of tests** • *Independent interpretation of a test performed by another physician/other qualified healthcare professional (not separately reported).* **or** **Category 3: Discussion of management or test interpretation** • *Discussion of management or test interpretation with external/physician/other qualified healthcare professional/appropriate source (not separately reported)*	*High risk of morbidity from additional diagnostic testing or treatment* Examples only: • *Drug therapy requiring intensive monitoring for toxicity* • *Decision for elective major surgery with identified patient or procedure risk factors* • *Decision for emergency major surgery* • *Decision regarding hospitalization* • *Decision for DNR or to de-escalate care because of poor prognosis* • *Parenteral controlled substances*

Table 6.42 Domiciliary, rest home, or custodial care services (established patient)

CC	*Burning with urination*
HPI	*76-year-old female states for 2 days she has had urgency and burning of urination; she does not have any abdominal pain or nausea or vomiting. States she has been eating and drinking well and does not feel she has had a fever.*
PFSH	*PMH- HTN, Diabetes type 2*
ROS	*General: does not report any chills* *Resp: does not report any shortness of breath* *Cardiac: does not report any chest pain* *Neuro: does report feeling weak and tired*
PE	*VS 135/76 p 92 4 18 t 99.1* *General: well appearing female in no acute distress* *Resp: lungs CTA* *Cardiac: RRR with no murmurs or rubs* *Abdomen: no CVA tenderness, slight suprapubic tenderness*
DIFF	*Simple UTI, complex UTI*
A/P	*Simple UTI: reviewed labs to see how her kidney function has been, prescribed macrodantin 100mg BID for 7 days, check BMP*
Time	*35 minutes spent reviewing records, examination of patient, documentation, review of ordered labs, and prescriptions.*

Table 6.43 Domiciliary, rest home, or custodial care services E/M coding

E/M code	History/Exam	MDM	Time
99347 – Established	*Clinician required to perform and document medically appropriate history and examination*	*Straightforward*	*Or 20 minutes*
99348 – Established		*Low*	*Or 35 minutes*
99349 – Established		*Moderate*	*Or 40 minutes*
99350 – Established		*High*	*Or 60 minutes*

MDM = 99348 Low

Time = 99348 Low

Table 6.44 Medical decision-making tool

MDM (2 out of 3 MDM)	Number of problems	Complexity of data reviewed	Risk of complications and or morbidity
Straightforward 99202 99212 99221 99231 99234	1 self-limited or minor problem	Minimal or NONE	Minimal risk of morbidity from additional diagnostic testing or treatment
Low complexity 99203 99213 99221 99231 99234	2 or more self-limited or minor problems **or** 1 stable, chronic illness **or** 1 acute uncomplicated illness or injury **or** 1 stable, acute illness **or** 1 acute, uncomplicated illness or injury requiring hospital inpatient or observation level of care	(Must meet 1 of 2 requirements of) **Category 1: Tests and documents** Any combination of 2 from the following • Review of prior external note(s) from each unique source • Review of the result(s) of each unique test • Ordering of each unique test **or** **Category 2: Assessment requiring an independent historian(s)**	Low risk of morbidity from additional diagnostic testing or treatment

Moderate	(Must meet 1 out of 3 requirements)	Moderate risk of morbidity from additional diagnostic testing or treatment
99204	**Category 1: Tests, documents, historian**	Examples only:
99214	*Any combination of 3 from the following*	
99222	• *Review of prior external note(s) from each unique source*	• *Prescription drug management*
99232	• *Review of the result(s) of each unique test*	• *Decision regarding minor surgery with identified patient or procedure risk factors*
99235	• *Ordering of each unique test*	
	• *Assessment requiring an independent historian(s)*	• *Decision regarding elective major surgery without identified patient or procedure risk factors*

1 or more chronic illnesses with exacerbation, progression, or side effects of treatment

or

2 or more stable chronic illnesses

or

1 undiagnosed new problem with uncertain prognosis

or

1 acute illness with systemic symptoms

or

1 acute, complicated injury

(Must meet 1 out of 3 requirements)

Category 1: Tests, documents, historian

Any combination of 3 from the following

• *Review of prior external note(s) from each unique source*

• *Review of the result(s) of each unique test*

• *Ordering of each unique test*

• *Assessment requiring an independent historian(s)*

or

Category 2: Independent interpretation of tests

• *Independent interpretation of a test performed by another physician/other qualified healthcare professional (not separately reported)*

or

Category 3: Discussion of management or test interpretation

• *Discussion of management or test interpretation with external/physician/ other qualified healthcare professional/appropriate source (not separately reported)*

Moderate risk of morbidity from additional diagnostic testing or treatment

Examples only:

• *Prescription drug management*

• *Decision regarding minor surgery with identified patient or procedure risk factors*

• *Decision regarding elective major surgery without identified patient or procedure risk factors*

• *Diagnosis or treatment significantly limited by social determinants of health*

(Continued)

Table 6.44 (Continued)

MDM (2 out of 3 MDM)	Number of problems	Complexity of data reviewed	Risk of complications and or morbidity
High complexity 99205 99215 99223 99233 99236	*1 or more chronic illnesses with severe exacerbation, progression, or side effects of treatment,* or *1 acute or chronic illness or injury that poses a threat to life or bodily function* or *Multiple morbidities requiring intensive management (Initial Nursing Facility only)*	*(Must meet 2 out of 3 requirements of)* **Category 1: Tests, documents, historian** *Any combination of 3 from the following* • *Review of prior external note(s) from each unique source* • *Review of the result(s) of each unique test* • *Ordering of each unique test* • *Assessment requiring an independent historian(s)* or **Category 2: Independent interpretation of tests** • *Independent interpretation of a test performed by another physician/other qualified healthcare professional (not separately reported)* or **Category 3: Discussion of management or test interpretation.** • *Discussion of management or test interpretation with external/physician/other qualified healthcare professional/appropriate source (not separately reported)*	*High risk of morbidity from additional diagnostic testing or treatment* Examples only: • *Drug therapy requiring intensive monitoring for toxicity* • *Decision for elective major surgery with identified patient or procedure risk factors* • *Decision for emergency major surgery* • *Decision regarding hospitalization* • *Decision for DNR or to de-escalate care because of poor prognosis* • *Parenteral controlled substances*

CRITICAL CARE SERVICES

Critical care codes are NOT being deleted and remain time-based (CPT 9921, 99292).

The definition of critical care remains the same:

An illness or injury that acutely impairs one or more vital organ systems such that there is a high probability of imminent of life-threatening deterioration in the patient's condition.

It involves decision making of high complexity to assess, manipulate and support vital organ system failure and / or to prevent further life-threatening deterioration of the patient's condition.

Example of vital organ systems include, but are not limited to

- Respiratory failure
- Circulatory failure
- Shock
- Renal, hepatic, metabolic failure
- Central nervous system failure

Critical care time must be:

- At the bedside
- On the unit and immediately available to patient
- Full attention
- May be aggregated
- Reviewing test results or imaging studies
- Discussing patient care with other medical staff
- Documented in the record
- Time spent with other decision makers when patient is unable to make decisions
- Time to perform procedures

Critical care time DOES NOT include time spent performing separately billed procedures. If you can answer YES to all 3 of the following questions you can count this as critical care time.

1. Is at least one vital organ system acutely impaired?
2. Is there a high probability of imminent, life-threatening deterioration?

3. Did you have to intervene to prevent further deterioration of the patient's condition?

A minimum of 30 minutes must be met to qualify for the initial CPT code, 99291.

You should document the exact minutes to exclude separately billed procedures.

Include in your documentation

- All differential diagnosis
- Which organ system is at risk
- What tests you ordered and why you ordered them or considered them
- In the emergency room, you would document all your reassessments and decision-making details
- Include the likelihood of life-threatening deterioration
- Document critical labs, imaging, EKG, or other findings that are of significance

ADDITIONAL SERVICES

PREVENTIVE MEDICINE COUNSELING

These codes are used when a NP or other qualified healthcare professional counsels the patient on lifestyle changes *prior to a specific illness* where you could consider the counseling a part of the treatment. Issues that could be addressed include family issues, diet and exercise, substance use, safe sexual practices, injury prevention, oral health counseling, and diagnostic and laboratory test results *if* they are available at the time of the visit. You would use **modifier 25** with your E/M code and then one of the following codes for the preventive service based on time.

For example, you are seeing an established patient for a chronic condition such as HTN that is controlled, and they are getting refills on their medication. You then spend an additional 15 minutes going over the labs that came in with the patient. For this example, you

Table 7.1 Additional codes for preventive medicine counseling

99201	*Approximately 15 minutes*
99402	*Approximately 30 minutes*
99403	*Approximately 45 minutes*
99404	*Approximately 60 minutes*

DOI: 10.4324/9781003542872-7

would calculate the E/M code for an established office patient, add modifier 25 and then 99201 for the extra 15 minutes you spent going over the labs.

PREVENTIVE BEHAVIOR COUNSELING

These codes are used when addressing a particular behavior. In these cases, the patient has an addiction or behavior that is deemed harmful such as tobacco use and addiction, vaping, substance abuse/misuse, or obesity. You may claim behavior change intervention for the following 3 reasons:

1. It is part of the treatment plan
2. The health condition is exacerbated by the behavior
3. Pre-emptively, prior to disease occurring such as smoking cessation prior to the development of COPD

For these codes you must document specific, validated interventions such as utilizing the Transtheoretical Stages of Change model to show *readiness for change*. Motivational interviewing techniques can be utilized to assist in *advising a change behavior* and assisting with *specific suggested actions*. Most providers take time to do these activities with their patients when a behavior poses a threat to a condition. By understanding the billing and coding rules you can capture payment for the services you are already delivering. With improved reimbursement you may be enabled to spend more time with your patients.

> **99406** – Smoking and tobacco cessation counseling must be greater than 3 minutes up to 10 minutes
> **99407** – Intensive greater than 10 minutes

> **99408** – ETOH or substance abuse structured screening (AUDIT, DAST) and brief intervention services – 15 to 30 minutes
> **99409** – Greater than 30 minutes

Only allocate one code at a visit: Either 99406 or 99407; Either 99408 or 99409

EXAMPLE NOTE (ESTABLISHED PATIENT)

CC: Shortness of breath

HPI: 58-year-old male with history of COPD has a 2-day history of increased shortness of breath with wheezing. Productive cough with yellow phlegm. States he is using his albuterol inhaler 4 times a day and finding it hard to catch his breath. Still smoking ½ pack per day cigarettes

Physical Exam: VS – 120/80 R 20 P 92 T 98.6

General: Well groomed, appears short of breath

Respiration: Wheezing bilaterally

Cardiac: RRR

Assessment and Plan: COPD exacerbation – DuoNeb's treatment, steroids, Rocephin 2 grams IM, Zithromax 500mg x 3 days, ordered CBC, and chest xray

Behavior Counseling: Discussed smoking cessation. Assessed patient's readiness to change utilizing the Stages of Change Model and patient is highly motivated to quit smoking. Utilizing motivational interviewing discussed ways in which patient felt that he has been successful in the past with smoking cessation. Pt feels that if he puts his cigarettes in an inconvenient place, he will be less likely to go get them because of the effort; this has worked in the past, and nicotine patches have also helped. He would like to pursue trying the patch again. **Time spent in counseling 10 minutes.**

For this example, you would calculate the E/M code for an established office patient – add modifier 25 and then 99307 for behavior counseling for smoking cessation.

ADVANCE CARE PLANNING

Use **99497** for the first 30 minutes you spend face-to-face with the patient, family member, and or surrogate to discuss advance directives such as standard forms with patient, family member, or surrogate by physician or qualified healthcare professional. Each additional 30 minutes requires code **99498**.

No active management of the problem(s) should take place during this conversation. 99497/99498 may be reported separately IF these services are performed on the SAME day as another evaluation and management service from the list below

- 99202–99215 Office visit or other outpatient service
- 99221–99223 Initial hospital inpatient or observation care
- 99231–99236 Subsequent hospital inpatient or observation care/admit/discharge same day
- 99238–99239 Hospital inpatient discharge
- 99242–99245 Office or other outpatient consultation
- 99252–99255 Inpatient or observation consultations
- 99281–99285 ER
- 99304–99310 Initial nursing facility care or subsequent nursing facility visits
- 99315–99316 Nursing facility discharge
- 99341–42; 99344–45 New home or residence services
- 99347–99350 Established home or residence services
- 99381–99397 Preventive services
- 99495–96 Transitional care management services

EXAMPLE: ADVANCE CARE PLANNING CONVERSATION

Pertinent Diagnosis: Altered mental status, UTI

Consent: The patient and/or family consented to a voluntary Advance Care Planning conversation. Individuals present for the conversation included the patient and husband.

Summary of the conversation: Code status addressed in which family states at this time he wants every life saving measure performed in the event of an emergency in which patient is unable to make a medical decision.

Outcome of the conversation and documents completed: Continue the current treatment plan and code status without modification.

Time: I spent 10 minutes providing separately identifiable ACP series with the patient and or surrogate decision maker in a voluntary, in-person conversation discussing the patient's wishes and goals as detailed in the above note.

MODIFIERS

CPT modifiers are codes that are used to either enhance or diminish a service without changing the procedural code. You add the modifier at the end of the CPT code separated by a dash. Here are some of the common modifiers you may use in practice.

- **Modifier 25** – on the same day a patient condition required a significant, separate identifiable D/M service, for example a significant problem is found during a well visit that requires further workup or preventive/behavioral counseling
- **Modifier 26** – professional component such as reading an xray
- **Modifier 32** – mandated service – such as a government-required service
- **Modifier 33** – preventive services – when the service is to deliver a USPST force preventive service A or B rating
- **Modifier 51** – multiple procedures
- **Modifier 57** – decision of surgery. An E/M service that results in a decision to perform surgery
- **Modifier 59** – different anatomic sites during same encounter such as lesions destroyed with cryotherapy

PROLONGED SERVICES

- **99417** Prolonged services approved by AMA which you can add on for every 15 minutes after the minimum time from a level on the date of an **office or other outpatient service, office**

consultation or other outpatient evaluation and management service (99205, 99215, 99245, 99345, 99350, 99483). For example, let's say you spent 75 minutes with a new office patient you would bill a 99205 (60 minutes) + 99417 (extra 15)

- **99418** Prolonged services approved by AMA which you can add on for every 15 minutes after the minimum time from a level on the date of an **inpatient evaluation and management service** (99223, 99233, 99236, 99255, 99306, 99310). For example, let's say you spent 65 minutes with an inpatient on a follow up visit you would bill a 99233 (50 minutes) + a 99217 (extra 15)

LEGAL IMPLICATIONS OF CODING AND BILLING

Fraud, waste, and abuse are significant issues in the American health-care system accounting for three percent annually or more than $300 billion of national healthcare spending (National Health Care Anti-Fraud Association [NHCAA], 2021). The Health Insurance Portability and Accountability Act of 1996 (HIPAA) established the national Health Care Fraud and Abuse Control Program (HCFAC) under the Attorney General and the Secretary of the Department of Health and Human Services (DHHS) to investigate, prosecute, and punish instances of systematic fraud and protect program beneficiaries. It is estimated that $4.7 billion annually is recovered under the False Claims Act (Furrow et al., 2018, p. 897).

While most providers regularly submit straightforward claims with documentation that supports coding and reflects accurate revenue and reimbursement, there are providers who yield to the appeal of higher revenue and reimbursement and exaggerate the complexity of services charged. Billing for services never performed and providing medical equipment that was not necessary are a few conspiracies alleged (Centers for Medicare and Medicaid Services [CMS], 2021). Cases of fraud, waste, and abuse are reported to DHHS or the Department of Justice (DOJ) by outside sources (i.e., whistleblowers), or discovered by internal or external audits, then processed for criminal prosecution and or civil actions (US Department of Health and Human Services, Office of Inspector General [USDHHS-OIG], n.d.).

DOI: 10.4324/9781003542872-8

Trust is foundational to the practitioner–patient relationship upon which quality care is built. Federal healthcare programs, including Medicare, rely on practitioners to make medical decisions that prioritize the welfare of patients while providing necessary care and services. The expectation is for practitioners to submit claims for payment that accurately reflect Medicare-covered items and services. However, fraudulent healthcare professionals who bill federal programs for personal gain must face laws that combat fraud, waste, and abuse, and safeguard appropriate medical care. NPs must comprehend the intricacies of medical coding and billing guidelines and federal fraud, waste, and abuse laws including the Anti-Kickback Statute, Stark Law, and False Claims Act, to uphold their professional integrity and ensure quality patient care.

ANTI-KICKBACK STATUTE (AKS)

The Anti-Kickback Statute is a law that attempts to protect patients from corrupt decision making for financial incentives between parties making healthcare decisions for them, including providers and suppliers (Furrow et al., 2018). Those incentives could be anything of value, any cash payments, loans, discounted rent or meals, free services, or other items of value, in effort to persuade or reward a referral to a federal healthcare program. When a provider offers incentives, or is reimbursed for, requests, or takes unauthorized compensation, the provider violates this law. As NPs become increasingly involved in the delivery of healthcare services, they must be aware of the legal implications of the AKS and how it applies to their practice. NPs cannot make payments, either directly or indirectly, for the purpose of inducing or rewarding a referral. For example, a NP cannot give a gift card to a patient in exchange for referring a friend or family member. NPs cannot accept payments, gifts, or other benefits from a third party in exchange for a referral.

In the $300 million healthcare fraud case, 11 defendants from Spectrum/Reliable pled guilty (Dooley, 2022). Ten defendants including two medical doctors and a NP were indicted on February 9, 2022, and an eleventh defendant charged on March 16, 2022. The defendants admitted paying and receiving illegal kickbacks to induce medical professionals to order medically unnecessary lab tests that were then billed to Medicare and other federal healthcare programs. As a result of the kickbacks, laboratories controlled by the defendants were able to submit more than $300 million in billing to federal government healthcare programs. The defendants, with charges ranging from conspiracy to concealment (misprison) of a felony, now face up to 15 years in federal prison.

NPs must be aware of the legal implications of the AKS and ensure that they abide by its provisions to avoid violations that can result in criminal and civil penalties, including fines, imprisonment, and exclusion (penalty as per the Exclusion Statute) from participating in Medicare and Medicaid programs. NPs may be subject to civil liability for damages, including treble damages and attorney's fees, if they are found to have violated the AKS. By understanding the AKS and its legal implications, NPs can help ensure that they are providing safe and ethical care to their patients.

STARK LAW

The Stark Law aims to protect patients and the resources of federal healthcare programs from conflicts of interest when a provider gains financially when making referrals for certain services that can be billed to Medicare by an entity in which that provider or a direct family member has ownership unless there is an exception (Furrow et al., 2018). Violations of the Stark Law can have serious legal and ethical consequences. Intentional or unintentional violations constitute overpayment that must be refunded within 60 days of being identified. Failure to make a refund is subject to a fine of $15,000 per item billed, treble damages, and exclusion from Medicare. In addition to the potential legal implications of violating the Stark Law, practitioners must also consider ethical implications as they are violating the patient's right to unbiased medical advice.

The Health Care Fraud and Abuse Control Program ([HCFAC]; USDHHS & DOJ, 2021) reports on the most egregious instances of healthcare fraud. In one case, several pain management clinics and a urine drug testing laboratory in South Carolina violated the Stark Law and the AKS for illegally incentivizing providers to refer patients for urine drug tests. They were required to pay over $136 million in civil False Claims Act (FCA) claims and over $4.2 million for billing federal healthcare programs for unnecessary urine drug tests. These fines are a result of the Civil Monetary Penalties Law (CMPL), an important tool for protecting the public, ensuring healthcare providers adhere to regulations, and determining monetary penalties based on the type of violation. While the penalties for violations of the law can be severe, understanding the law and the potential consequences of violating it can help providers remain in compliance and avoid the costly penalties associated with non-compliance.

The Stark Law applies to NPs in the same way as it does to physicians. NPs may not receive any payment from an entity to which they refer a Medicare or Medicaid patient, and they may not receive any direct or indirect payment for such a referral. Additionally, NPs may not refer a patient to a facility or service in which they have a financial interest. If a NP does have a financial interest in a facility or service, they must disclose this to the patient before any referral is made. NPs must be aware of the requirements of the law, as well as the ethical implications of making referrals based on financial gain.

FALSE CLAIMS ACT (FCA)

False Claims Act (FCA) violations occur when a false claim is intentionally submitted to collect federal money. The FCA protects the federal government from being fleeced or sold inferior products or services. Under this act, providers can be held accountable for civil penalties from $10,781 to $21,563 per claim along with additional treble charges or three times the damages incurred (Furrow et al., 2018). The FCA also has incentives for individuals (whistleblowers) to report fraud and the misuse of government funds and provides strong legal remedies for those who are found guilty.

In one case, a NP in Florida was sentenced to 12 months and 1 day in prison and ordered to pay $23,880,678 in restitution after pleading guilty to conspiring to solicit and receive illegal kickbacks and executing a healthcare fraud scheme. The NP received illegal kickbacks from telemedicine and other companies to sign orders and prescriptions for medically unnecessary items, including DME, genetic testing, and prescription medications. The NP did not have a prior provider–patient relationship with these patients and did not evaluate or assess their needs. Patients were solicited through media ads and cold calls, and their insurance information was obtained.

The NP received numerous complaints from patients, yet the federal healthcare benefit programs paid $23,880,678 for the fraudulent orders and prescriptions signed by the NP between 2017 and 2019.

NPs are a vital part of the healthcare system and must adhere to the same rules and regulations as other healthcare professionals when it comes to billing for services provided. This includes complying with the FCA. Failure to comply with the FCA can result in severe financial penalties, including hefty fines and even imprisonment. Filing false claims can be considered fraud, which is a criminal offense, and can lead to criminal charges, as well as other disciplinary actions, such as the loss of license or certification. NPs must protect themselves by becoming familiar with the law, staying up to date on any changes that may occur, ensure that they are in compliance with all applicable laws and regulations, and accurately and honestly document all services provided. NPs should closely review all claims for reimbursement before submitting them to the government. NPs must adhere to the law and understand the potential legal repercussions of violating the FCA.

UPCODING AND UNDER CODING

Healthcare fraud committed by providers exploits helpless or unwitting patients and violates the oath they took to protect patients. Ultimately, a provider's financial arrangements with federal and state healthcare programs, including Medicare and Medicaid, are subject to laws aimed to prevent over and underutilization of healthcare services and recoup funds paid based on fraudulent claims. Violations that result in overbilling, under-billing, fraud, and abuse are discoverable through audits by the DOJ who work to preserve the integrity of public health programs and prevent improper billing practices. When providers boost their profits by billing federal healthcare programs for more expensive services than needed, the Office of Inspector General (OIG) will ensure they are held accountable for their deceptive schemes settling disputes using fines and or jail time.

UPCODING

Upcoding is the practice of submitting claims for reimbursement for services provided to patients that are higher than the actual services provided. For example, evaluation and management (E/M) codes may be misused to up code an established patient at a higher-level E/M code. Also, upcoding may include the misuse of the modifier 25 – allowing additional payment for a medically unnecessary E/M service (CMS, 2021). The consequences for upcoding are serious ranging from civil penalties that include hefty fines and repayment of overbilled amounts, to criminal penalties that include jail time. Due to their increasing role in patient care, NPs are more likely to be exposed to upcoding and are at a greater risk of upcoding when working with billing staff or when they are unfamiliar with billing codes or coding systems. It is important for NPs to have a thorough understanding of billing codes and coding systems to ensure that they are providing accurate information when submitting claims for reimbursement.

In the case brought forth by a whistleblower lawsuit, the DOJ, District of Massachusetts Attorney General accused CareWell of submitting false claims to Medicare, Massachusetts Medicaid (MassHealth), Massachusetts Group Insurance Commission (GIC), and Rhode Island Medicaid by inflating and upcoding the level of E/M services performed and failing to properly identify the providers of E/M services (DOJ, 2021). CareWell allegedly mandated medical personnel to examine and document at least 13 body systems during medical history inquiries and at least nine body systems during physical examinations, even if patients' specific medical complaints did not justify such comprehensive inquiries or examinations. CareWell also allegedly used encounter plan templates, loaded onto electronic medical records software, containing "yes or no" questions that CareWell directed its personnel to ask patients regarding specific body systems, even when such inquiries were not medically necessary. The government alleged that CareWell failed to reduce the amounts of its claims to Medicare, MassHealth, GIC, and Rhode Island Medicaid for services performed by unsupervised NPs. The accusations suggest a calculated scheme by CareWell to unjustly benefit from government healthcare resources.

"Inflating bills and submitting claims to government health insurance programs for needless services drains resources from legitimate patient care. Those seeking to enrich themselves at the expense of these taxpayer-funded programs must be held accountable" (DOJ, 2021, para. 6). Whistleblower lawsuits filed under the *qui tam* provisions of the FCA permit private individuals to sue on behalf of the government for false claims and share in any monetary financial recovery.

To reduce risk and protect themselves from legal liability, NPs should learn about the billing codes and coding systems and should ensure that all claims submitted for reimbursement accurately reflect the services provided to the patient.

UNDER CODING

The Centers for Medicare and Medicaid Services (CMS, 2021) offer a fact sheet on Medicare Fraud and Abuse, which doesn't mention "under coding" specifically but implies it as a compliance risk. Under coding could be considered a violation of fraud and abuse rules as it involves misrepresenting services provided. Deliberate under coding is "making a false statement" about the services provided and "knowingly billing for services that were not furnished" and "misusing codes on a claim" for under coding would be considered fraud and abuse, respectively. Also, under the Criminal Health Care Fraud statute (CMS, 2021), it is a crime to "obtain (by means of false or fraudulent pretenses, representations, or promises) any of the money or property owned by, or under the custody or control of, any health care benefit program" (p. 10). Under coding could also lead to false utilization patterns and flag a provider as an outlier, making them a target for investigation and audits. For example, consider the Anti-Kickback Statute, coding services at lower than actual levels might be interpreted as an inducement to patients (who could benefit by having a lower co-pay).

Under coding can be a controversial and complicated subject, especially when it comes to the role of a NP in the healthcare system. NPs are responsible for accurately coding patient visits and submitting claims to insurance companies. Down coding can result in fraud charges, fines, and even jail time, therefore, it is important for NPs to be aware of the potential legal implications of down coding and to make sure they are complying with all applicable regulations.

ADVICE

The "legal analysis" of coding and billing for the most part has gone unchanged for the last 30 years and providers are encouraged to create practices with compliance programs, self-audits, and checks for exclusions that reduce instances of healthcare fraud and abuse (Buppert, 2021). Further, because E/M codes are financially tied to documentation practices, it is essential that providers accurately bill, code, and complete self-audits (quarterly, annually) that can detect and prevent fraud, waste, and abuse. Violations to acceptable standard coding and billing practices result in investigation.

Following clinical practice guidelines and medical coding can enable NPs to access ethical billing processes using standard codes. Medicare, as well as other payors, use standard procedure and diagnosis codes to ensure the items billed merit the procedures, tests, or treatments. Practitioners and those with designated specialties must follow these basic rules for coding (CMS, 2022):

- Practitioners should only report documented procedures
- Practitioners should report procedure and diagnosis codes in sequence
- Practitioners should follow National Correct Coding Initiatives (NCCI) and

Medical Unlikely Edits (MUE)

- Practitioners should become familiar with any new coding changes throughout the year

NP SERVICES

Insurance companies may have additional requirements for billing that can change over time. It is a good idea for practitioners to check with insurance companies to ensure they meet the necessary requirements for billing their services. Practitioners should follow these general service requirements (CMS, 2022):

- The NP is legally authorized to practice in the state where services are furnished (Buppert, 2021)
- Reasonable and necessary services are not statutorily precluded; services are considered physician services if a medical doctor or doctor of osteopathy provided them
- NP services are provided in collaboration with a physician
- NP assistant-at-surgery services may be covered

- Services and supplies are furnished *incident to* NP professional services provided
- NP supervision of other non–physicians does not constitute a personal professional performance of that service

NP BILLING

Billing practices may vary depending on the state or region therefore it is important to check with relevant authorities and insurance companies to ensure appropriate guidelines are being followed. Practitioners should follow these general billing practices (CMS, 2022):

- Directly bill for services using their NPI
- Allow an employer or contractor to use their NPI to bill reassigned services
- Bill using the supervising physician's NPI *incident to* professional services provided by the NP
- Use the NP's NPI to bill services provided *incident to* their own professional services
- Bill assistant-at-surgery services and report only the AS modifier on the claim form
- Provide services on an assignment-related basis but not charge a patient more than the amounts permitted under 42 CFR 424.55
- Refund payment to the patient if they paid for a service over these limits

NP PAYMENT

Payment guidelines for NPs may vary depending on the state and region in which they practice. It is always a good idea for NPs to familiarize themselves with payment models (fee for service, salary, capitation) and reimbursement rates in their region. Practitioners should follow these general payment guidelines (CMS, 2022):

- Payment is only on assignment i.e., pre-approved amount
- Payment is 80% of the lesser of the actual charge or 85% of the amount the physician gets under the Medicare physician fee schedule (PFS)

- Direct payment is provided for assistant-at-surgery services at 85% of 16% of the amount a physician receives under the Medicare PFS
- Payment for services provided incident to an NP outside a hospital setting is 85% of the amount a physician gets under the Medicare PFS
- Payment for hospital inpatient and outpatient services is unbundled and directly furnished to the NP
- Payment for professional services is furnished only when the NP performs the services and there is no facility or provider charges
- Payment is not provided to other professionals for providing services

Taking time upfront to code and bill each patient encounter correctly will assure that you are doing the best job that you can to prevent improperly processed claims. In other words, applying the coding rules to billable services and using supporting medical necessity documented in the medical record will promote those rules and demonstrate fiscal responsibility to providers, payers, and patients. Comporting oneself professionally and following accepted coding practices are in your best interest and reflect that you have the patient's and payer's best interests at heart (Buppert, 2021).

Patients may have a poor relationship with their provider yet if they had a rapport with their provider, a higher level of trust may be realized. Establishing a good provider–patient relationship may be as simple as not rushing patients, being more engaging in conversation, understanding the patient's medical, social, and mental history, and being open to questions. It is important to take time with patients because they may require a trusting, long-term relationship with you as their provider. Patients may also express heightened awareness of how financial factors affect the healthcare system. These factors make patients more skeptical of the care they are receiving and therefore depend upon providers to invest more in establishing relationships built on trust and shared decision making.

Finally, it is important to stay informed of fraud and abuse laws, and prevent or report violations such as upcoding, under coding, and violations of AKB and Stark Law because providers and the insurance industry profit from these violations (CMS, 2021).

Additionally, the new direct contracting entities (DCEs) are accelerating the privatization of Medicare, treating healthcare as a profit-making commodity rather than a social need (Strether, 2021). Become proactive and contact your state and federal elected representatives to address these issues and other concerns including supporting HR 1976 (Congress.gov, 2021), a federal bill that aims to bring affordable, comprehensive medical care to everyone without the corrupting effects of profit-making entities.

The high cost of healthcare is a barrier to care for many low-income patients, who are at increased risk of financial harm from unnecessary tests and treatments that offer little to no benefit. This can reinforce fears that providers may be influenced by factors other than the patient's best interests, such as incentives from pharmaceutical companies or reimbursement levels from insurance companies. Yet, patients are more informed today regarding potential conflicts of interest in the healthcare system and may feel the need to guard against providers' potential conflicts of interest. Providers should also be mindful that marginalized populations and communities of color, who have a distrust of being deliberately harmed by the healthcare system, now have greater access, a stronger voice, and expect systems of injustice replaced with trust building healthcare systems that address public health core values (equity, social justice, affordability, accessibility), structural competency and transparency within institutions, and awareness of structural barriers and systemic racism (Best et al., 2022).

REFERENCES

Best, A. L., Fletcher, F. E., Kadono, M., & Warren, R. C. (2022). Institutional distrust among African Americans and building trustworthiness in the COVID-19 response: Implications for ethical public health practice. *Journal of Health Care for the Poor and Underserved, 32*(1), 90–98. Retrieved from https://www.ncbi.nlm.nih.gov/pmc/articles/PMC7988507/

Buppert, C. (2021). *Nurse practitioner's business practice and legal guide* (7th ed.). Jones and Bartlett Learning.

Centers for Medicare and Medicaid Services (CMS). (2022). Advanced practice registered nurses, anesthesiologist assistants, and physician assistants. Retrieved from https://www.cms.gov/Outreach-and-Education/Medicare-Learning-Network-MLN/MLNProducts/Downloads/Medicare-Information-for-APRNs-AAs-PAs-Booklet-ICN-901623.pdf

CMS. (2021). Medicare fraud & abuse: Prevent, detect, report. Retrieved from https://www.cms.gov/Outreach-and-Education/Medicare-Learning-Network-MLN/MLNProducts/Downloads/Fraud-Abuse-MLN4649244.pdf

Congress.gov. (2021). HR 1976 Medicare for All Act of 2021. Retrieved from https://www.congress.gov/bill/117th-congress/house-bill/1976

Department of Justice, United States Attorney's Office, District of Massachusetts. (2021). CareWell Urgent Care Center agrees to pay $2 million to resolve allegations of false billing of government health care programs. Retrieved from https://www.justice.gov/usao-ma/pr/carewell-urgent-care-center-agrees-pay-2-million-resolve-allegations-false-billing

Dooley, E. (2022). 11 defendants plead guilty in $300 million healthcare fraud. United States Attorney's Office, Northern District of Texas. Retrieved from https://www.justice.gov/usao-ndtx/pr/11-defendants-plead-guilty-300-million-healthcare-fraud

Furrow, B. R., Greaney, T. L., Johnson, S. H., Stoltzfus-Jost, T., Schwartz, R. L., Clark, B. R., Fuse-Brown, E. C., Gatter, R., King, J. S., & Pendo, E. (2018). *Health law cases, materials, and problems* (8th ed.). West Academic Publishing.

National Health Care Anti-Fraud Association (NHCAFA). (2021). *The challenge of healthcare fraud*. Retrieved from https://www.nhcaa.org/tools-insights/about-health-care-fraud/the-challenge-of-health-care-fraud/

Strether, L. (2021). Direct contracting entities: The latest scam to privatize Medicare. *Physicians for National Health Program (PNHP)*. Retrieved from https://pnhp.org/news/direct-contracting-entities-the-latest-scam-to-privatize-medicare/

US Department of Health and Human Services (USDHHS), Office of Inspector General [USDHHS-OIG]. (n.d.). Whistleblower protection coordinator. Retrieved from https://oig.hhs.gov/fraud/whistleblower/

USDHHS & US Department of Justice (DOJ). (2021). Health care fraud and abuse control program annual report for fiscal year 2021. Retrieved from https://oig.hhs.gov/publications/docs/hcfac/FY2021-hcfac.pdf

9

MEDICAL NECESSITY

"Medical necessity" is a legal doctrine in the United States defined by Title XVII of the Social Security Act, 1862[a][1][A] as an item or service that is "reasonable and necessary for the diagnosis and treatment of illness or injury or to improve the functioning of a malformed body member." Inseparable from this legal statute is the notion that items and services provided must satisfy standards of medical practice, patient safety, contractual scope, medical service and or setting, and costs. Ideally, providers consult books and journals on a day-to-day basis, regularly attend continuing education presentations, make referrals to specialists when necessary, and seek consultation when necessary to avert practice errors (Buppert, 2021). Below are common factors associated with medical necessity:

- Clinical judgment
- Chief complaint
- Acute exacerbations/onset of medical conditions or injury
- Stability or acuity of patient
- Multiple medical co-morbidities
- Management of patient for that specific day of service (DOS)
- Professional standards applied to the symptoms, diagnosis, and treatment of the condition, illness, disease, or injury

DOI: 10.4324/9781003542872-9

Medical necessity is supported by the chief complaint, yet a chronic condition alone does not meet medical necessity. Below are common observations associated with medical necessity:

- Medical necessity is used as criterion for payment
- Reimbursement by Medicare is not required when the visit is mandated by the state or facility, unless the visit is medically necessary
- Volume of documentation does not determine the evaluation and management (E/M) level that is coded
- Provider documentation should clearly explain medical necessity in the plan of care noting how the visit has or will change the patient's health outcomes

Medical necessity cases must reflect a well-established, generally accepted standard in the medical community otherwise allegations of fraud (medically unnecessary care) or negligence can be launched. Consider the following examples of medical necessity and the complexities surrounding each case.

EXAMPLE I

For each provider–patient encounter, documentation must show that the levels of history, exam, and MDM performed are medically necessary and include tests and therapeutic interventions ordered or performed. Consider the following case of an established patient who presents with a chief complaint of intermittent chest pain with occasional shortness of breath. A comprehensive history shows location, severity, duration of chest pain, modifying factors, and associated signs and symptoms. The patient's past medical history (PMH) reveals risk factors i.e., coronary artery disease (CAD), hypertension (HTN), and dyslipidemia (DLP). A family history reveals cardiovascular disease (CD), and a social history reveals smoking and sedentary lifestyle. A complete 8-system physical exam is justified to obtain a definitive diagnosis and treatment plan. An abnormal EKG at the office visit warrants an immediate cardiac catheterization for suspected CAD. The patient has diabetes (DM), HTN, and is on anti-coagulation therapy that requires adjustment prior to the procedure. A comprehensive history, comprehensive examination, and medical decision making (MDM) of high complexity support the code of 99215 for this encounter. In the 1995 or 1997 Documentation

Guidelines for Established Patients, two of the three components of history, an exam, and the MDM *were* met; in the current guidelines the complexity of MDM alone would also justify this level of care.

If a denial in payment for medical necessity is received, it may be the result of missing documentation and or the appropriate application of codes with/without modifiers. If medical necessity is not apparent from the provider–patient encounter, then the claim will not be reimbursed no matter how severe the patient's condition or how complicated the provider's thought process. Medical necessity and MDM are not the same. MDM refers to the complexity of making a diagnosis and selecting a management option. Medical necessity refers to the appropriateness of the service provided for a condition. In other words, medical necessity determines whether the provider's service will receive reimbursement.

EXAMPLE II

Quality of care involves preserving health and restoring health when injury occurs through the work of healthcare providers, facilities, and interrelated services. Practice guidelines establish a foundation for standard of care, offering recommendations, yet guidelines can be altered to fit the needs of a particular patient (Furrow et al., 2018). Consider the case of a provider who followed practice guidelines as the standard of care. In the 1974 case of Helling v. Carey, Carey did not test Helling, who was symptomatic for glaucoma, citing that the medical standards for the testing of glaucoma were for patients older than age 40; Helling was younger than 40 (Standard, 2019). Helling, who was later diagnosed with glaucoma, sued Carey alleging that permanent damage to the eye was due to failure of an early diagnosis and treatment. The trial and appeals courts sided with Carey but the Supreme Court sided with Helling finding Carey negligent. Even when following the standard of care, if the symptoms were there, then Carey should have tested for glaucoma using a simple pressure test. While practice guidelines published by medical associations i.e., American Academy of Ophthalmology ([AAO], 2024) or governmental bodies (Medicare.gov) direct and reimburse care that is reasonable and medically necessary for the diagnosis and treatment of an illness, disease, or its symptoms, the provider is ultimately responsible for tailoring their approach when a unique health condition presents itself in order to justify a variance from the standard of care.

Rigid adherence to guidelines may not be in the patient's best interest as guidelines are designed to guide routine care but emphasize clinical judgment when patients present with specific symptoms. These important elements align with clinical judgment and medical management, and contribute to high-quality care.

EXAMPLE III

To increase the rate of the use of appropriate advanced diagnostic imaging services and reduce the risk of cancer from radiation exposure, Section 218(b) of the Protecting Access to Medicare Act ([PAMA]; CMS, 2022a) of 2014 requires an ordering provider (OP) to utilize the appropriate use criteria (AUC) accessible through qualified clinical decision support mechanisms ([CDSMs]; Centers for Medicare and Medicaid Services [CMS], 2022a, 2022c). AUCs and CDSMs are endorsed by CMS and typically appear imbedded within the electronic medical record (EHRs) or can be easily accessed through website-based portals. As of January 1, 2021, OPs must consult AUCs for all advanced diagnostic imaging services – computed tomography (CTs), magnetic resonance imaging (MRI), nuclear medicine, and positron emission tomography (PET) scans (American College of Radiology, 2020). When a patient receives an initial CT scan, the exposure contains 25mSv with 8 years of background radiation. This same patient may receive a second CT scan doubling exposure, background radiation, and increasing their risk for cancer. AUCs serve as a guideline for practice standards on medically necessary imaging and support the OP in their efforts to reduce patient exposure to radiation. Exceptions to use of AUCs include treating patients in emergency services, inpatient settings, and critical access hospitals, and for OPs experiencing significant hardship i.e., lack of EHRs with CDSMs. AUCs are currently utilized for traditional Medicare patients, not Medicare Advantage patients, and include G-codes and modifiers.

These three cases illustrate the use of objective scientific evidence to determine medical necessity. Yet, in the case where harm occurred, prosecution triggered increased scrutiny on clinical judgment. The threat of prosecution for medical necessity is entirely avoidable when alternatives are considered rather than using standards/criteria for a coverage decision.

MEANINGFUL USE

In 2012, CMS introduced the meaningful use (MU) of health information to bring higher-quality care, improve patient safety (reduce medical errors), show how big data can reveal the most effective treatments, and empower patients with their own portable medical record (CMS, 2022c). Providers who received financial reimbursement demonstrated meaningful use of certified EHRs, met core and menu set objectives, and reported quality measures to CMS (CMS, 2022b). EHRs made it easy to identify patterns, locate hidden problems that are fixable (detect inappropriate care, improve compliance), spot trends (improve checklists for discharge planning, timely prescribing for best outcomes) and monitor outliers (address upcoding practices). After 2015, incentive payments changed to payment reductions for those providers who did not demonstrate MU. Today 96% of hospitals and 86% of provider practices have adopted EHRs.

EHRs were supposed to save $81 billion dollars per year yet led to software failures and the realization that digitizing health information to streamline care would be problematic and unreliable (Schulte & Fry, 2019). Additionally, the framers of the EHR financial incentive programs discovered perverse business dynamics of technology companies who placed 'gag clauses' to discourage providers from speaking out on the safety issues and technology failures to avoid litigation. With respect to a host of risks to patient safety created by EHRs, near misses, serious injuries, and alarming reports of deaths due to system flaws or user errors have remained in repositories, never compiled for analysis or opportunities to improve safety (Schulte & Fry, 2019). Consider the following example of MU and the complexities surrounding the case.

HOW MEANINGFUL USE CAN FAIL

EHR legal pitfalls and threats to providing care that is medically necessary occur when providers experience a high number of electronic notifications and ignore them due to being overwhelmed, also known as alert fatigue. Consider this provider who ordered Prednisone 120 mg every other day for renal failure however the nurse sent the prescription as daily to the pharmacy. Several alerts were sent to the provider. The provider approved without looking at the alert. The nurse reinforced that the correct prescription was ordered by checking what the nurse sent not what the physician ordered. The patient's caregiver alerted the healthcare provider of this high dose and was again reassured that the prescription was correct. The patient presented for a procedure nine days later with complaints of tremors, esophageal burning, hiccups, stomach pain, and swallowing problems. On day eight, the patient had called the provider not feeling well and was told to reduce Prednisone to 10 mg daily. The patient was diagnosed with hypotension and tachycardia, went to the hospital and died two days later. The autopsy showed angio invasive gram positive microorganisms, multiple ulcers of the colon with full penetration through the muscular wall, peritonitis, and interstitial lung fibrosis (Buppert, 2021).

Today's provider spends half of their day or more clicking through menus and typing rather than interacting with patients. If providers could work smarter, harder, and longer to improve the system they would have already done so. Ashish Jha et al. (2019), White House Coronavirus Response Coordinator in 2024, blames much of provider burnout on the cognitive burden from navigating poorly designed EHRs and performing tasks that do not directly benefit the patient. While the age of paper charting had its errors (misinterpreting the practitioner's writing, documenting in the wrong chart), todays EHR errors (poor interface designs i.e., missed lab orders, typed notes disappearing) create moral injury. Moral injury is a profound and unrecognized threat to one's wellbeing because of a broken healthcare system where providers are unable to consistently meet patients' needs and remain wounded, disengaged, and increasingly hopeless (Damania, 2019; Dean et al., 2019).

QUALITY

Consumer groups, like the National Committee for Quality Assurance (NCQA), compare managed care plans on performance measures (health outcomes, access to providers) and patient satisfaction to compel providers to evaluate their performance, use of services, and quality care (Buppert, 2021). In other words, providers must demonstrate appropriate treatment, record a rational explanation of the visit, code and bill for appropriate reimbursement, track and trend outcomes, and utilize data to improve performance and reduce healthcare costs. Ultimately, medical necessity is the overarching criterion that connects these various forces to ensure payment upfront and avoid the time-consuming denial and appeal processes on the back end.

STATE RESPONSIBILITIES

States are responsible for providing access, utilization, and quality care for medically necessary services, for example, to Medicaid enrollees under age 21 that include screening, vision, dental, hearing, diagnostic, and other necessary healthcare services, along with treatment (Early and Periodic Screening, Diagnostic, and Treatment [EPSDT], 2022). EPSDT (2022) benefits include guides and strategies (care coordination, mental health, oral health, well-care visits) to increase efficiency and effectiveness of care for children under age 21 who depend on Medicaid for their health. Optimal EPSDT benefits can be realized when barriers are addressed that affect access to services, supply of providers, presence of managed care, linguistic and disability access, and transportation.

Medicare reimbursement is contingent on whether an item or service fits with a statutory benefit category, is not excluded from coverage, and is reasonable and necessary. Medical necessity can be managed prospectively, concurrently (as part of the workflow to support care decisions), or retroactively and is based on national coverage determination ([NCDs]; CMS, 2022d). NCDs grant, limit, or exclude Medicare coverage for an item or service and encourage the public to participate in determining coverage for an item or service. For example, the Medicare Evidence Development and Coverage Advisory Committee (MEDCAC) reviews an item or service under the Social Security Act and debates the benefits i.e., pulmonary pressure sensor for heart failure management, the competence level of the provider, and requirements of the facility before an item or service is considered reasonable or necessary and added as a covered item or service. As an example of politics in healthcare policy, during the Biden Administration, CMS removed 298 procedures on the inpatient only (IPO) list, reversing a proposed rule by the Trump Administration. Further, CMS codified the removal of procedures making it clear in regulatory text that only CMS will evaluate future procedures for removal (Trotter, 2021). The reversal of hundreds of outpatient surgeries left businesses frustrated who cancelled plans to build outpatient surgery centers ([OSC]; Zipp, 2021).

LOOKING FORWARD

What can NPs expect? No provider should expect to be sued for a poor outcome when there was no actual malpractice on the part of the provider. NPs should stay informed, become an advocate for patients, and get politically involved. Take the extra time with dissatisfied patients, involve risk management, and attempt to resolve problems (long waits, impersonal treatment, busy signals when calling the office) to defuse potential lawsuits (Buppert, 2021).

Expect to be regulated for documenting medical necessity that reflects appropriate services and accurate codes. CMS posts regulatory changes on the Federal Register. Providers and vendors can provide their comments before the final rule. These commentaries inform regulators how the proposed changes do or do not support the provider's clinical practice. Providers can support or reject the proposed changes, but their comments are a matter of public record and the final rule posted and published must be followed (Federal Register, 2022). Regulatory changes may originate from provider and vendor proposals requesting to update the international disease classification (ICD-10) and statistical manual of mental disorders (DSM-5) coding systems based on new scientific advances. The American Medical Association (AMA) and the American Psychiatric Association (APA) websites contain proposal forms to request changes and information on updated codes. The AMA link to request CPT changes is:

https://www.ama-assn.org/about/cpt-editorial-panel/cpt-code-process

The APA link for proposal requests on ICD-10 codes is:

https://www.psychiatry.org/psychiatrists/practice/dsm/submit-proposals

Expect state and or federal legislation to drive provider compliance on practice standards i.e., utilizing AUCs accessible through CDSMs prior to ordering diagnostic imaging services. Expect provider and insurance data to be tracked, monitored, and rewarded or penalized. Expect hedge fund and private equity firms to invest in health technology, addiction treatment services, and acquire provider practices and infiltrate chronically under-resourced cultures, degrade the healthcare delivery system, and take advantage of clinician professionalism (Gustafsson et al., 2019). Their risky business model of buying to improve efficiency, then abruptly shutting down healthcare systems for a handsome profit is problematic and unsustainable (Gale, 2020a; Tribble, 2022).

Healthcare spending receives 19.7% of the nation's Gross Domestic Product (GDP), reaching $4.1 trillion or $12,530 per person. These regrettably high healthcare costs have to do with how the medical industrial complex (insurance industry, pharmaceutical companies, hospitals) can charge as much as they want, legally. Despite spending more than other countries, the Organization for Economic Co-operation Development (OECD), *who compares industrialized nations' healthcare spending for policy improvement and for better health outcomes*, reported a stark increase in spending from 9.3% (1983) to 16.8% (2019) and projects spending $6.2 trillion by 2028; and there is no sign of slowing down (Schneider et al., 2021).

Make time for politics. Expect politics to play a larger role in the business of healthcare especially when addressing social determinants of health i.e., access to affordable, accessible healthcare. Has your state implemented Medicaid expansion? (Kaiser Family Foundation [KFF], 2022). Proposals to counter the rising cost of US healthcare expenditures include policies related to price transparency to promote competition (Makary, 2021; Scott et al., 2022) and a single payer system. Physicians for National Health Care (PNHC) along with other professional organizations have supported *Medicare for All*. While *Medicare for All* may be politically unpopular, having one payment system would consolidate fragmented finances, improve resource allocation, and reduce waste (Weisbart, 2012).

The price of healthcare is notoriously inflated. It's a monopoly pure and simple and studies have shown hospitals were paid more than double what Medicare paid for the same services (Gordon, 2022). Research shows there is no correlation between price and outcome (Gale, 2020b). As of July 1, 2022, CMS issued the Transparency in Coverage Final Rule that requires healthcare insurers to disclose prices for covered services and items. This follows the January 1, 2022 implementation of the No Surprises Act that protects patients from unexpected, predatory charges for certain services. It may take a while for payers to follow the new rulings and benefits to materialize. In a cautionary tale from the January 1, 2021 Hospital Price Transparency Final Rule, only 14% of hospitals are in compliance (Gordon, 2022). Finally, inform your patients that you are on their side and expose unfair charging for items and services by sending patients to Dr. Rosenthal's Bill of the Month website at Kaiser Health News ([KHN], 2022). Dr. Rosenthal examines hospitals bills and the hospital's charge master, then helps reduce patients' hospital bills significantly. These strategies can help protect the integrity of your role as a NP and help patients survive medical billing!

REFERENCES

American Academy of Ophthalmology. (2024). Guideline central. Retrieved from https://www.guidelinecentral.com/guidelines/AAO/

American College of Radiology. (2020). 2020 Annual report. Retrieved from https://www.acr.org/About-ACR/Annual-Reports/2020-Annual-Report

Buppert, C. (2021). *Nurse practitioner's business practice and legal guide* (7th ed.). Jones and Bartlett Learning.

Centers for Medicare and Medicaid Services (CMS). (2022a). Appropriate use criteria program. CMS.gov. Retrieved from https://www.cms.gov/Medicare/Quality-Initiatives-Patient-Assessment-Instruments/Appropriate-Use-Criteria-Program

CMS. (2022b). General frequently asked questions. Retrieved from https://www.cms.gov/Regulations-and-Guidance/Legislation/EHRIncentive-Programs/Downloads/FAQ_General.pdf

CMS. (2022c). Appropriate use criteria program. CMS.gov. Retrieved from https://www.cms.gov/Medicare/Quality-Initiatives-Patient-Assessment-Instruments/Appropriate-Use-Criteria-Program

CMS. (2022d). Medicare coverage determination process. https://www.cms.gov/Medicare/Coverage/DeterminationProcess

Damania, Z. (2019). It's not burnout, it's moral injury. ZDOGGMD. https://zdoggmd.com/moral-injury/

Dean, W., Talbot, S., & Dean, A. (2019). Reframing clinician distress: Moral injury not burnout. *Federal Practitioner*, 36(9). Retrieved from https://www.ncbi.nlm.nih.gov/pmc/articles/PMC6752815/

Early and Periodic Screening, Diagnostic, and Treatment. (2022, August 15). Medicaid.gov.

Federal Register. (2022). https://www.federalregister.gov/index/2022

Furrow, B. R., Greaney, T. L., Johnson, S. H., Stoltzfus Jost, T., Schwartz, R. L., Clark, B. R., Fuse Brown, E. C., Gatter, R., King, J. S., & Pendo, E. (2018). *Health law: Cases, materials, and problems* (8th ed.). West Academic Publishing.

Gale, A. H. (2020a). I stuffed their mouths with gold part II. *Missouri Medicine, 117*(4), 296–298.

Gale, A. H. (2020b). The price we pay – What broke American health care and how to fix it. *Missouri Medicine, 117*(1), 18–19.

Gordon, D. (2022, July 3). New healthcare price transparency rule took effect July 1, but it may not help much yet. *Forbes*. https://www.forbes.com/sites/debgordon/2022/07/03/new-healthcare-price-transparency-rule-took-effect-july-1-but-it-may-not-help-much-yet/?sh=27dfffda8e72

Gustafsson, L., Seervai, S., & Blumenthal, D. (2019, October, 19). The role of private equity in driving up health care prices. *Harvard Business Review*. https://hbr.org/2019/10/the-role-of-private-equity-in-driving-up-health-care-prices

Jha, A. K., Iliff, A. R., Chaoui, A. A., Defossez, S., Bombaugh, M. C., & Miller, Y. R. (2019). A crisis in health care: A call to action on physician burnout. https://cdn1.sph.harvard.edu/wp-content/uploads/sites/21/2019/01/PhysicianBurnoutReport2018FINAL.pdf

Kaiser Family Foundation (KFF). (2022, July 21). Status of state Medicaid expansion decisions: Interactive map. Retrieved from https://www.kff.org/medicaid/issue-brief/status-of-state-medicaid-expansion-decisions-interactive-map/

Kaiser Health News. (2022). *Bill of the month.* https://khn.org/news/tag/bill-of-the-month/

Makary, M. (2021). *The price we pay: What broke American health care and how to fix it.* Bloomsbury Publishing, Inc.

Medicare.gov (2024). Is your test, item, or service covered? Medicare.gov Retrieved from https://www.medicare.gov/coverage/is-your-test-item-or-service-covered

Schneider, E. C., Shah, A., Doty, M. M., Tikkanen, R., Fields, K., & Williams II, R. D. (2021). Mirror, mirror 2021: Reflecting poorly. Healthcare in the US compared to other high income countries. *The Commonwealth Fund.* https://www.commonwealthfund.org/publications/fund-reports/2021/aug/mirror-mirror-2021-reflecting-poorly

Schulte, F. & Fry, Erika. (2019). Death by 1,000 clicks: Where electronic health records went wrong. KHN. Retrieved from https://khn.org/news/death-by-a-thousand-clicks/

Scott, M. P., Clemon, D., & Kvilhaug, S. (2022). Why U. healthcare spending is rising so fast. *Investopedia.* https://www.investopedia.com/u-s-healthcare-spending-rising-fast-5186172

Social Security. *Compilation of the social security laws.* (2022). Retrieved from https://www.ssa.gov/OP_Home/ssact/title18/1862.htm

Standard of care. (2019, March 20). *Legal dictionary.* Retrieved from https://legaldictionary.net/standard-of-care/

Tribble, S. J. (2022). Buy and bust. When private equity comes for rural hospitals. *Kaiser Health News.* Retrieved from https://khn.org/news/article/private-equity-rural-hospitals-closure-missouri-noble-health/

Trotter, Z. (2021). CMS reverses course on elimination of the inpatient-only service list. *Waller.* https://www.wallerlaw.com/news-insights/3956/CMS-reverses-course-on-elimination-of-the-inpatient-only-service-list-

Weisbart, E. (2012). A single payer system would reduce US healthcare costs. *AMA Journal of Ethics,* 14(11), 897–903. https://journalofethics.ama-assn.org/article/single-payer-system-would-reduce-us-health-care-costs/2012-11

Zipp, R. (2021, November 3). CMS reinstates Medicare's inpatient only list in final rule, reversing Trump era nix. MedTechDive. Retrieved from https://www.medtechdive.com/news/cms-restores-ipo-list-medtronic-stryker/609367/

PRACTICE CODING

OFFICE VISIT

Example 1.1 New patient office visit

CC   *Establish care*

HPI   *76-year-old female with c/o abdominal pain x 1 week in*
       RUQ – seems to occur after eating a fatty meal. Pt states attacks
       are painful and rates pain 7 out of 10. Nothing seems to make
       them better just avoiding certain foods.

PFSH *Obesity, HTN, HLD*

ROS   *Constitution: denies weight gain or loss*
       Resp: denies SOB
       Cardiac: denies chest pain/palpitations/syncope
       Abdominal: c/o urgent diarrhea after meals at times

PE   *Constitutional: VS 130/80 p 99 r 16, appears well*
       HR: regular heartbeat noted, no edema
       Respiration: CTA with normal respiratory effort
       GI: RUQ tenderness with positive Murphy's sign

(Continued)

DOI: 10.4324/9781003542872-10

Example 1.1 (Continued)

CC	*Establish care*

A/P *Possible cholecystitis – ordered RUQ ultrasound, CBC, CMP*
HTN: stable at goal of < 140/80 continue same meds
HLD: Lipids reviewed from previous practice and are at goal of < 100;
  continue statin

TIME *45 minutes (review of records, examination of patient, completing*
  documentation and placing orders)

Example 1.2 E/M codes for new patient office visits

E/M code	History/Exam	MDM	Time
99202	Clinician required to perform and document medically appropriate history and examination	Straightforward	Or 15–29
99203		Low complexity	Or 30–44
99204		Mod complexity	Or 45–59
99205		High complexity	Or 60–74

MDM =

Time =

Example 1.3 Medical decision-making tool

MDM (2 out of 3 MDM)	Number of problems	Complexity of data reviewed	Risk of complications and or morbidity
Straightforward			
99202	*1 self-limited or minor problem*	*Minimal or NONE*	*Minimal risk of morbidity from additional diagnostic testing or treatment*
99212			
99221			
99231			
99234			
Low complexity			
99203	*2 or more self-limited or minor problems*	*(Must meet 1 of 2 requirements)*	*Low risk of morbidity from additional diagnostic testing or treatment*
99213	***or***	**Category 1: Tests and documents**	
99221	*1 stable, chronic illness*	*Any combination of 2 from the following*	
99231	***or***	• *Review of prior external note(s) from each unique source*	
99234	*1 acute uncomplicated illness or injury*	• *Review of the result(s) of each unique test*	
	or	• *Ordering of each unique test*	
	1 stable, acute illness	***or***	
	or	**Category 2: Assessment requiring an independent historian(s)**	
	1 acute, uncomplicated illness or injury requiring hospital inpatient or observation level of care		

| **Moderate**
99204
99214
99222
99232
99235 | 1 or more chronic illnesses with exacerbation, progression, or side effects of treatment
or
2 or more stable chronic illnesses
or
1 undiagnosed new problem with uncertain prognosis
or
1 acute illness with systemic symptoms
or
1 acute, complicated injury | *(Must meet 1 out of 3 requirements)*
Category 1: Tests, documents, historian
Any combination of 3 from the following
• *Review of prior external note(s) from each unique source*
• *Review of the result(s) of each unique test*
• *Ordering of each unique test*
• *Assessment requiring an independent historian(s)*
or
Category 2: Independent interpretation of tests
• *Independent interpretation of a test performed by another physician/ other qualified healthcare professional (not separately reported).* | *Moderate risk of morbidity from additional diagnostic testing or treatment*
Examples only:
• *Prescription drug management*
• *Decision regarding minor surgery with identified patient or procedure risk factors*
• *Decision regarding elective major surgery without identified patient or procedure risk factors*
• *Diagnosis or treatment significantly limited by social determinants of health* |

(Continued)

Example 1.3 (Continued)

MDM (2 out of 3 MDM)	Number of problems	Complexity of data reviewed	Risk of complications and or morbidity
		or	
		Category 3: Discussion of management or test interpretation	
		• Discussion of management or test interpretation with external/ other qualified physician/ other qualified healthcare professional/appropriate source (not separately reported)	
High complexity	1 or more chronic illnesses with severe exacerbation, progression, or side effects of treatment	*(Must meet 2 out of 3 requirements of)* **Category 1: Tests, documents, historian** Any combination of 3 from the following:	High risk of morbidity from additional diagnostic testing or treatment
99205			
99215		• Review of prior external note(s) from each unique source	Examples only:
99223	*or*	• Review of the result(s) of each unique test	• Drug therapy requiring intensive monitoring for toxicity
99233	1 acute or chronic illness or injury that poses a threat to life or bodily function	• Ordering of each unique test	
99236		• Assessment requiring an independent historian(s)	• Decision for elective major surgery with identified patient or procedure risk factors
	or		
	Multiple morbidities requiring intensive management (Initial Nursing Facility only)		

or

Category 2: Independent interpretation of tests

- *Independent interpretation of a test performed by another physician/ other qualified healthcare professional (not separately reported)*

or

Category 3: Discussion of management or test interpretation

- *Discussion of management or test interpretation with external/ physician/ other qualified healthcare professional/appropriate source (not separately reported)*

- *Decision for emergency major surgery*
- *Decision regarding hospitalization*
- *Decision for DNR or to de-escalate care because of poor prognosis*
- *Parenteral controlled substances*

Example 2.1 Established patient office visit

CC	*c/o left knee pain*
HPI	*12-year-old playing basketball at school reports acute pain in left knee after abrupt turn. States it hurts to bear weight. Rates pain as 10 out of 10*
PFSH	
ROS	
PE	*Constitutional: VS 130/90 p 88 R 16 Weight 98 pounds*
	Cardiac: RRR no murmurs
	Skin: Warm and dry
	Extremity: left knee with effusion; Apley maneuver positive, difficult to bear weight
	CT scan shows meniscal tear
A/P	*1. Left knee meniscus tear: knee brace, pain rx, refer to ortho (spoke with orthopedist) school note given for no GYM*
TIME	*45 minutes (review of records, examination of patient, discussion with mother, documentation, and preparation of discharge paperwork to include prescription)*

Example 2.2 E/M codes for established patient office visit

E/M code	History/Exam	MDM	Time
99211	Clinician required to perform and document medically appropriate history and examination	None	NA
99212		Straightforward	Or 10–19
99213		Low complexity	Or 20–29
99214		Mod complexity	Or 30–39
99215		High complexity	Or 40–54

MDM =

TIME =

Example 2.3 Medical decision-making tool

MDM (2 out of 3 MDM)	Number of problems	Complexity of data reviewed	Risk of complications and or morbidity
Straightforward			
99202 99212 99221 99231 99234	*1 self-limited or minor problem*	*Minimal or NONE*	*Minimal risk of morbidity from additional diagnostic testing or treatment*
Low complexity	*2 or more self-limited or minor problems*	*(Must meet 1 of 2 requirements)*	*Low risk of morbidity from additional diagnostic testing or treatment*
99203 99213 99221 99231 99234	*or* *1 stable, chronic illness* *or* *1 acute uncomplicated illness or injury* *or* *1 stable, acute illness* *or* *1 acute, uncomplicated illness or injury requiring hospital inpatient or observation level of care*	**Category 1: Tests and documents** *Any combination of 2 from the following* • *Review of prior external note(s) from each unique source* • *Review of the result(s) of each unique test* • *Ordering of each unique test* *or* **Category 2: Assessment requiring an independent historian(s)**	

(Continued)

Example 2.3 (Continued)

MDM (2 out of 3 MDM)	Number of problems	Complexity of data reviewed	Risk of complications and or morbidity
Moderate 99204 99214 99222 99232 99235	1 or more chronic illnesses with exacerbation, progression, or side effects of treatment **or** 2 or more stable chronic illnesses **or** 1 undiagnosed new problem with uncertain prognosis **or** 1 acute illness with systemic symptoms **or** 1 acute, complicated injury	*(Must meet requirements of 1 out of 3)* **Category 1: Tests, documents, historian** Any combination of 3 from the following • Review of prior external note(s) from each unique source • Review of the result(s) of each unique test • Ordering of each unique test • Assessment requiring an independent historian(s) **or** **Category 2: Independent interpretation of tests** • Independent interpretation of a test performed by another physician/other qualified healthcare professional (not separately reported) **or** **Category 3: Discussion of management or test interpretation** • Discussion of management or test interpretation with external/physician/ other qualified healthcare professional/appropriate source (not separately reported)	Moderate risk of morbidity from additional diagnostic testing or treatment Examples only: • Prescription drug management • Decision regarding minor surgery with identified patient or procedure risk factors • Decision regarding elective major surgery without identified patient or procedure risk factors • Diagnosis or treatment significantly limited by social determinants of health

High complexity

99205
99215
99223
99233
99236

1 or more chronic illnesses with severe exacerbation, progression, or side effects of treatment, **or** 1 acute or chronic illness or injury that poses a threat to life or bodily function **or** Multiple morbidities requiring intensive management (Initial Nursing Facility only)	(Must meet 2 out of 3 requirements of) **Category 1: Tests, documents, historian** Any combination of 3 from the following • Review of prior external note(s) from each unique source • Review of the result(s) of each unique test • Ordering of each unique test • Assessment requiring an independent historian(s) **or** **Category 2: Independent interpretation of tests** • Independent interpretation of a test performed by another physician/other qualified healthcare professional (not separately reported) **or** **Category 3: Discussion of management or test interpretation** • Discussion of management or test interpretation with external/physician/other qualified healthcare professional/appropriate source (not separately reported)	High risk of morbidity from additional diagnostic testing or treatment Examples only: • Drug therapy requiring intensive monitoring for toxicity • Decision for elective major surgery with identified patient or procedure risk factors • Decision for emergency major surgery • Decision regarding hospitalization • Decision for DNR or to de-escalate care because of poor prognosis • Parenteral controlled substances

ACUTE CARE

Example 3.1 Inpatient or initial observation

CC	*SOB*
HPI	*65 yo female with c/o increasing SOB over past 2 days. Pt normally does not wear oxygen now requiring 4L per nasal cannula. c/o weight gain of 10 pounds over past 3 days with ankle swelling. States she now must sleep on 3 pillows and cannot walk across her living room without resting.*
PFSH	*PMH HTN* *Soc hx smokes 1 ppd for past 50 years*
ROS	*Constitution: c/o weight gain of 10 pounds in last 3 days* *Lungs: c/o increased SOB with orthopnea* *Cardiac: denies any chest pressure or palpitations, states her ankles have been swollen*
PE	*VS 180/80 p 88 r 20* *Constitution: alert in minimal distress* *Resp: obvious WOB cannot complete sentences, Lungs with bilateral rales* *Cardiac: RRR no murmurs, 2 + pedal edema*
DIFF	*CHF exacerbation, Pulmonary embolism, Pneumonia*
Provider	*Spoke with ER physician to admit; spoke with cardiology*
A/P	*1. New onset Systolic decompensated CHF − reviewed CXR which was normal − pro BNP was 35,000 up from 17,000 last admit 6 months ago; reviewed Echo done 6 months ago by cardiologist, and she had a normal EF of 75% at that time; will start Lasix 40 mg IV BID, monitor daily BMP, consult cardiology, admit to telemetry, and repeat Echo* *2. HTN urgency − as evidenced by elevated BP 1870/80 and CKD with GFR of 35 − resume home meds and add hydralazine 50mg TID*
TIME	*45 minutes (review of records, examination of patient, coordination of care and documentation including orders)*

Example 3.2 Initial observation and inpatient E/M service codes

E/M code	History/ Exam	MDM	Time
99221	Clinician required to perform and document medically appropriate history and examination	Straightforward or Low	Or 40 minutes
99222		Moderate	Or 55 minutes
99223		High	Or 75 minutes

MDM =

Time =

Example 3.3 Medical decision-making tool

MDM (2 out of 3 MDM)	Number of problems	Complexity of data reviewed	Risk of complications and or morbidity
Straight forward 99202 99212 99221 99231 99234	*1 self-limited or minor problem*	*Minimal or NONE*	*Minimal risk of morbidity from additional diagnostic testing or treatment*
Low complexity 99203 99213 99221 99231 99234	*2 or more self-limited or minor problems* **or** *1 stable, chronic illness* **or** *1 acute uncomplicated illness or injury* **or** *1 stable, acute illness* **or** *1 acute, uncomplicated illness or injury requiring hospital inpatient or observation level of care*	*(Must meet 1 of 2 requirements)* **Category 1: Tests and documents** *Any combination of 2 from the following* • *Review of prior external note(s) from each unique source** • *Review of the result(s) of each unique test** • *Ordering of each unique test** **or** **Category 2: Assessment requiring an independent historian(s)**	*Low risk of morbidity from additional diagnostic testing or treatment*

Moderate

99204
99214
99222
99232
99235

1 or more chronic illnesses with exacerbation, progression, or side effects of treatment

or

2 or more stable chronic illnesses

or

1 undiagnosed new problem with uncertain prognosis

or

1 acute illness with systemic symptoms

or

1 acute, complicated injury

(Must meet 1 out of 3 requirements)

Category 1: Tests, documents, historian

Any combination of 3 from the following

- Review of prior external note(s) from each unique source*
- Review of the result(s) of each unique test*
- Ordering of each unique test*
- Assessment requiring an independent historian(s)

or

Category 2: Independent interpretation of tests

- Independent interpretation of a test performed by another physician/other qualified healthcare professional (not separately reported)

or

Category 3: Discussion of management or test interpretation

- Discussion of management or test interpretation with external/physician/other qualified healthcare professional/appropriate source (not separately reported)

Moderate risk of morbidity from additional diagnostic testing or treatment

Examples only:

- Prescription drug management
- Decision regarding minor surgery with identified patient or procedure risk factors
- Decision regarding elective major surgery without identified patient or procedure risk factors
- Diagnosis or treatment significantly limited by social determinants of health

(Continued)

Example 3-3 (Continued)

MDM (2 out of 3 MDM)	Number of problems	Complexity of data reviewed	Risk of complications and or morbidity
High complexity 99205 99215 99223 99233 99236	*1 or more chronic illnesses with severe exacerbation, progression, or side effects of treatment* or *1 acute or chronic illness or injury that poses a threat to life or bodily function* or *Multiple morbidities requiring intensive management (Initial Nursing Facility only)*	*(Must meet 2 out of 3 requirements)* **Category 1: Tests, documents, historian** *Any combination of 3 from the following* • *Review of prior external note(s) from each unique source** • *Review of the result(s) of each unique test** • *Ordering of each unique test** • *Assessment requiring an independent historian(s)* or **Category 2: Independent interpretation of tests** • *Independent interpretation of a test performed by another physician/other qualified healthcare professional (not separately reported)* or **Category 3: Discussion of management or test interpretation** • *Discussion of management or test interpretation with external/physician/ other qualified healthcare professional/appropriate source (not separately reported)*	*High risk of morbidity from additional diagnostic testing or treatment* Examples only: • *Drug therapy requiring intensive monitoring for toxicity* • *Decision for elective major surgery with identified patient or procedure risk factors* • *Decision for emergency major surgery* • *Decision regarding hospitalization* • *Decision for DNR or to de-escalate care because of poor prognosis* • *Parenteral controlled substances*

Example 4.1 Subsequent hospital inpatient and observation services (progress note)

CC	**Back pain**
HPI	*73 yo female pt was admitted for acute back pain x 3 days after coughing fit. Xray shows compression fracture at L3/4. Rates pain 7 out of 10, unable to walk without severe pain*
Interval change	*Vertebroplasty performed; rates pain as 3 out of 10*
PE	*Constitutional – alert x3, appears well*
	Muscular skeletal – unsteady gait, walking slowly, normal muscle strength and tone
	Neurological – DTR in lower extremities normal, normal sensation
Provider	*Ortho has seen patient and has no further interventions planned*
A/P	*1. Compression fracture: PT/OT recommending SNF for rehab – walked 20 feet with walker and SBA, requiring pain rx, start volteran cream TID*
TIME	*20 minutes (review of records, examination of patient, coordination of care and documentation including orders)*

Example 4.2 Subsequent observation and inpatient service E/M codes

E/M code	History/Exam	MDM	Time
99231	*Clinician required to perform and document medically appropriate history and examination*	*Straightforward or low*	*Or 25 minutes*
99232		*Moderate*	*Or 35 minutes*
99233		*High*	*Or 50 minutes*

MDM =

Time =

Example 4-3 Medical decision-making tool

MDM (2 out of 3 MDM)	Number of problems	Complexity of data reviewed	Risk of complications and or morbidity
Straight forward 99202 99212 99221 99231 99234	*1 self-limited or minor problem*	*Minimal or NONE*	*Minimal risk of morbidity from additional diagnostic testing or treatment*
Low complexity 99203 99213 99221 99231 99234	*2 or more self-limited or minor problems* *or* *1 stable, chronic illness* *or* *1 acute uncomplicated illness or injury* *or* *1 stable, acute illness* *or* *1 acute, uncomplicated illness or injury requiring hospital inpatient or observation level of care*	*(Must meet 1 of 2 requirements)* **Category 1: Tests and documents** *Any combination of 2 from the following* • *Review of prior external note(s) from each unique source* • *Review of the result(s) of each unique test* • *Ordering of each unique test* *or* **Category 2: Assessment requiring an independent historian(s)**	*Low risk of morbidity from additional diagnostic testing or treatment*

Moderate

99204
99214
99222
99232
99235

1 or more chronic illnesses with exacerbation, progression, or side effects of treatment

or

2 or more stable chronic illnesses

or

1 undiagnosed new problem with uncertain prognosis

or

1 acute illness with systemic symptoms

or

1 acute, complicated injury

(Must meet 1 out of 3 requirements)

Category 1: Tests, documents, historian

Any combination of 3 from the following
- Review of prior external note(s) from each unique source
- Review of the result(s) of each unique test
- Ordering of each unique test
- Assessment requiring an independent historian(s)

or

Category 2: Independent interpretation of tests
- Independent interpretation of a test performed by another physician/other qualified healthcare professional (not separately reported)

or

Category 3: Discussion of management or test interpretation
- Discussion of management or test interpretation with external/physician/other qualified healthcare professional/appropriate source (not separately reported)

Moderate risk of morbidity from additional diagnostic testing or treatment

Examples only:

- *Prescription drug management*
- *Decision regarding minor surgery With identified patient or procedure risk factors*
- *Decision regarding elective major surgery without identified patient or procedure risk factors*
- *Diagnosis or treatment significantly limited by social determinants of health*

(Continued)

Example 4.3 (Continued)

MDM (2 out of 3 MDM)	Number of problems	Complexity of data reviewed	Risk of complications and or morbidity
High complexity 99205 99215 99223 99233 99236	*1 or more chronic illnesses with severe exacerbation, progression, or side effects of treatment* *or* *1 acute or chronic illness or injury that poses a threat to life or bodily function* *or* *Multiple morbidities requiring intensive management (Initial Nursing Facility only)*	*(Must meet 2 out of 3 requirements)* **Category 1: Tests, documents, historian** *Any combination of 3 from the following* • *Review of prior external note(s) from each unique source* • *Review of the result(s) of each unique test* • *Ordering of each unique test* • *Assessment requiring an independent historian(s)* *or* **Category 2: Independent interpretation of tests** • *Independent interpretation of a test performed by another physician/other qualified healthcare professional (not separately reported)* *or* **Category 3: Discussion of management or test interpretation** • *Discussion of management or test interpretation with external/physician/other qualified healthcare professional/appropriate source (not separately reported)*	*High risk of morbidity from additional diagnostic testing or treatment* Examples only: • *Drug therapy requiring intensive monitoring for toxicity* • *Decision for elective major surgery with identified patient or procedure risk factors* • *Decision for emergency major surgery* • *Decision regarding hospitalization* • *Decision for DNR or to de-escalate care because of poor prognosis* • *Parenteral controlled substances*

Example 5.1 Admit/discharge same day

CC	*Abdominal pain*
HPI	**17 yo female with 1 day h/o epigastric abdominal pain that has been increasing. Pt states it is knifelike. Rates severity 8 out of 10. Movement makes it worse; nothing seems to make it better.**
PFSH	*No sig PMH*
ROS	*C/o feeling feverish; c/o RLQ abdominal pain as per HPI* *c/o nausea*
PE	*VS 100/80 76 16, appears unwell* *ENT: nares patent with no drainage, no posterior pharynx erythema* *Resp: CTA bilaterally – normal respiratory effort* *Cardiac: RRR-, no pedal edema* *Abd: guarded with positive McBurney, positive heel-jar* *Skin: warm and dry* *CT of abdomen shows acute appendicitis* *WBC count 18,000*
DIFF	*Acute appendicitis; Pelvic inflammatory disease; acute gallbladder disease; ectopic pregnancy, ovarian cyst*
Provider	*Accepted patient from ER; Spoke with surgeon after procedure*
Admission Dx	*Acute Appendicitis*
Discharge Dx	*Acute Appendicitis s/p lab appendectomy*
Dispo	*Home*
Code status	*Full*
Condition	*Good*
Discharge instructions	*No heavy lifting x1 week, no tub baths for 1 week; PRN Percocet given for pain; as well as Colace 100mg BID*
TIME	*65 minutes*

Example 5.2 Admit/DC same day observation and inpatient E/M service codes

E/M code	History/Exam	MDM	Time
99234	Clinician required to perform and document medically appropriate history and examination	Straightforward or low	Or 40 minutes
99235		Moderate	Or 70 minutes
99236		High	Or 85 minutes

MDM =

Time =

Example 5.3 Medical decision-making tool

MDM (2 out of 3 MDM)	Number of problems	Complexity of data reviewed	Risk of complications and or morbidity
Straight forward 99202 99212 99221 99231 99234	1 self-limited or minor problem	Minimal or NONE	Minimal risk of morbidity from additional diagnostic testing or treatment
Low complexity 99203 or 99213 99221 or 99231 99234	2 or more self-limited or minor problems or 1 stable, chronic illness or 1 acute uncomplicated illness or injury or 1 stable, acute illness or 1 acute, uncomplicated illness or injury requiring hospital inpatient or observation level of care	(Must meet 1 of 2 requirements) **Category 1: Tests and documents** Any combination of 2 from the following • Review of prior external note(s) from each unique source • Review of the result(s) of each unique test • Ordering of each unique test or **Category 2: Assessment requiring an independent historian(s)**	Low risk of morbidity from additional diagnostic testing or treatment

(Continued)

Example 5.3 (Continued)

MDM (2 out of 3 MDM)	Number of problems	Complexity of data reviewed	Risk of complications and or morbidity
Moderate 99204 99214 99222 99232 99235	*1 or more chronic illnesses with exacerbation, progression, or side effects of treatment* **or** *2 or more stable chronic illnesses* **or** *1 undiagnosed new problem with uncertain prognosis* **or** *1 acute illness with systemic symptoms* **or** *1 acute, complicated injury*	*(Must meet 1 out of 3 requirements)* **Category 1: Tests, documents, historian** *Any combination of 3 from the following* • *Review of prior external note(s) from each unique source* • *Review of the result(s) of each unique test* • *Ordering of each unique test* • *Assessment requiring an independent historian(s)* **or** **Category 2: Independent interpretation of tests** • *Independent interpretation of a test performed by another physician/other qualified healthcare professional (not separately reported)* **or** **Category 3: Discussion of management or test interpretation** • *Discussion of management or test interpretation with external/physician/ other qualified health care professional/ appropriate source (not separately reported)*	*Moderate risk of morbidity from additional diagnostic testing or treatment* Examples only: • *Prescription drug management* • *Decision regarding minor surgery with identified patient or procedure risk factors* • *Decision regarding elective major surgery without identified patient or procedure risk factors* • *Diagnosis or treatment significantly limited by social determinants of health*

High complexity	1 or more chronic illnesses with severe exacerbation, progression, or side effects of treatment **or** 1 acute or chronic illness or injury that poses a threat to life or bodily function **or** Multiple morbidities requiring intensive management (Initial Nursing Facility only)	**or**	*(Must meet 2 out of 3 requirements)* **Category 1: Tests, documents, historian** Any combination of 3 from the following • Review of prior external note(s) from each unique source • Review of the result(s) of each unique test • Ordering of each unique test • Assessment requiring an independent historian(s) **Category 2: Independent interpretation of tests** • Independent interpretation of a test performed by another physician/other qualified healthcare professional (not separately reported) **or** **Category 3: Discussion of management or test interpretation** • Discussion of management or test interpretation with external/physician/other qualified healthcare professional/appropriate source (not separately reported)	*High risk of morbidity from additional diagnostic testing or treatment* Examples only: • Drug therapy requiring intensive monitoring for toxicity • Decision for elective major surgery with identified patient or procedure risk factors • Decision for emergency major surgery • Decision regarding hospitalization • Decision for DNR or to de-escalate care because of poor prognosis • Parenteral controlled substances
99205 99215 99223 99233 99236				

HOSPITAL DISCHARGE

Example 6.1 Hospital discharge note

Day of admission	5/2/2022
Day of discharge	5/4/2022
Discharge diagnosis	Chest pain – noncardiac Muscle strain
Brief physical exam	• alert x3 • cardiac – RRR • Resp – CTA • Skin – warm and dry
Hospital course	48-year-old male admitted with c/o exertional chest pain. Rated pain a 7 out of 10. Cardiac markers x3 neg, EKG normal. Stress test did not show signs of ischemia. Pt pain improved with Toradol. Normal kidney function.
Discharge meds	None; may take OTC Motrin or Aleve for pain, use Volteran cream QID
Additional tests	No further tests needed
Follow up	f/u with primary care doctor in 7 days
Dispo	Home
Condition	Good
Code	Full
Time	Total time spent in review of record, physical exam, coordination of care with care givers and preparation of discharge paperwork is __ 35 minutes

Example 6.2 Hospital discharge day management E/M coding

E/M code	Face-to-face encounter	Time
99238	Clinician required to perform and document medically appropriate history and examination	≤ 30 minutes
99239		≥ 30 minutes

Time =

Example 7.1 Emergency room

CC	*Complaint of left ear pain*
HPI	*8-month-old infant with c/o pulling on left ear, crying when laid down, fever x1 day. Max temp in last 24 hours 102.6 under arm, improved with ibuprofen*
PFSH	*No significant PMH; parents do smoke in the house*
ROS	• *Constitution: mother reports max temp 102.6* • *ENT: Mother reports pulling on left ear, mother reports some clear nasal drainage* • *GI: Mother denies decreased appetite, vomiting or diarrhea*
PE	• *Constitution: T 103 P 90 R 16, fussy* • *ENT: Left TM bulging with fluid in middle ear, nares with clear drainage, posterior pharynx red with petechial rash on pillars* • *Resp: CTA bilaterally* • *Skin: warm, dry, no rash*
DIFF	*Otitis Media; Serous Otitis Media; Viral Pharyngitis; Strep Pharyngitis*
Provider	*NA*
Testing	**Strep test positive**
Dx	*1. Strep throat − per rapid test − prescribed amoxicillin* *2. Left acute OM − on higher dose of amoxicillin for 10 days*
Discharge instructions	*Complete all antibiotics; return to PCP or clinic if no improvement in next 24 hours*
Time	*24 minutes*

Example 7.2 Emergency room E/M coding

E/M code	History/Exam	MDM
99281	*Clinician required to perform and document medically appropriate history and examination*	*N/A*
99282		*Straightforward*
99283		*Low*
99284		*Moderate*
99285		*High*

MDM = 99283 Low

NO TIME COMPONENT

Example 7.3 Medical decision-making tool

MDM (2 out of 3 MDM)	Number of problems	Complexity of data reviewed	Risk of complications and or morbidity
Straightforward 99202 99212 99221 99231 99234	1 self-limited or minor problem	Minimal or NONE	Minimal risk of morbidity from additional diagnostic testing or treatment
Low complexity 99203 99213 99221 99231 99234	2 or more self-limited or minor problems or 1 stable, chronic illness or 1 acute uncomplicated illness or injury or 1 stable, acute illness or 1 acute, uncomplicated illness or injury requiring hospital inpatient or observation level of care	(Must meet 1 of 2 requirements) **Category 1: Tests and documents** Any combination of 2 from the following • Review of prior external note(s) from each unique source* • Review of the result(s) of each unique test* • Ordering of each unique test* or **Category 2: Assessment requiring an independent historian(s)**	Low risk of morbidity from additional diagnostic testing or treatment

Moderate

99204
99214
99222
99232
99235

1 or more chronic illnesses with exacerbation, progression, or side effects of treatment

or

2 or more stable chronic illnesses

or

1 undiagnosed new problem with uncertain prognosis

or

1 acute illness with systemic symptoms

or

1 acute, complicated injury

(Must meet 1 out of 3 requirements)

Category 1: Tests, documents, historian

Any combination of 3 from the following

- Review of prior external note(s) from each unique source*
- Review of the result(s) of each unique test*
- Ordering of each unique test*
- Assessment requiring an independent historian(s)

or

Category 2: Independent interpretation of tests

- Independent interpretation of a test performed by another physician/other qualified healthcare professional (not separately reported)

orç

Category 3: Discussion of management or test interpretation

- Discussion of management or test interpretation with external/physician/other qualified healthcare professional/appropriate source (not separately reported)

Moderate risk of morbidity from additional diagnostic testing or treatment

Examples only:

- Prescription drug management
- Decision regarding minor surgery with identified patient or procedure risk factors
- Decision regarding elective major surgery without identified patient or procedure risk factors
- Diagnosis or treatment significantly limited by social determinants of health

(Continued)

Example 7.3 (Continued)

MDM (2 out of 3 MDM)	Number of problems	Complexity of data reviewed	Risk of complications and or morbidity
High complexity 99205 99215 99223 99233 99236	*1 or more chronic illnesses with severe exacerbation, progression, or side effects of treatment* **or** *1 acute or chronic illness or injury that poses a threat to life or bodily function* **or** *Multiple morbidities requiring intensive management (Initial Nursing Facility only)*	*(Must meet 2 out of 3 requirements of)* **Category 1: Tests, documents, historian** *Any combination of 3 from the following* • *Review of prior external note(s) from each unique source** • *Review of the result(s) of each unique test** • *Ordering of each unique test** • *Assessment requiring an independent historian(s)* **or** **Category 2: Independent interpretation of tests** • *Independent interpretation of a test performed by another physician/other qualified healthcare professional (not separately reported)* **or** **Category 3: Discussion of management or test interpretation** • *Discussion of management or test interpretation with external/physician/other qualified healthcare professional/appropriate source (not separately reported)*	*High risk of morbidity from additional diagnostic testing or treatment* Examples only: • *Drug therapy requiring intensive monitoring for toxicity* • *Decision for elective major surgery with identified patient or procedure risk factors* • *Decision for emergency major surgery* • *Decision regarding hospitalization* • *Decision for DNR or to de-escalate care because of poor prognosis* • *Parenteral controlled substances*

SKILLED NURSING FACILITY SERVICES

Example 8.1 Skilled Nursing Facility services: Initial visit

CC	*Failing to thrive*
HPI	*86 yo female with failure to thrive. Comes from hospital with decreased appetite and loss of 20 pounds past several months, w/u did not reveal underlying cause.*
PFSH	*PMH HTN, HLD, DM type 2, Depression, Macular degeneration, Covid 19 3 months ago* *Fam hx — parents deceased* *Soc hx — denies smoking, ETOH socially*
ROS	• *Constitution: c/o fatigue* • *Resp: denies SOB, DOE, or orthopnea* • *Cardiac: denies CP or palpitations* • *GI: c/o no appetite since COVID; occasional diarrhea* • *Psychiatric: c/o lack of interest in activities*
PE	• *Constitution: VS 120/80 P 80 R 20 weight 98 pounds* • *Respiratory: decreased breath sounds bilaterally* • *Cardiac: RRR no murmurs, thrills; no edema* • *Skin: warm and dry without rashes* • *Psyc: good insight and judgment: PHQ 9 15 (moderate depression)*
A/P	• *Review and summation of old records* • *Long Haul Covid — continue nebs* • *Depression — start Remeron 7.5mg nightly* • *HTN — under good control continue Lisinopril/ HCTZ* • *DM type 2 — HgA1c — diabetic diet — continue metformin*
TIME	*Total time spent 55 minutes in review of hospital records, examination of patient, finalization of admission orders to include medication reconciliation, and ordering of lab work.*

Example 8.2 E/M codes for Initial Nursing Facility services

E/M Code	History/Exam	MDM	Time
99304	Clinician required to perform and document medically appropriate history and examination	Straightforward or low	Or 25 minutes
99305		Moderate	Or 35 minutes
99306		High	Or 45 minutes

MDM =

Time =

Example 8.3 Medical decision-making tool

MDM (2 out of 3 MDM)	Number of problems	Complexity of data reviewed	Risk of complications and or morbidity
Straightforward			
99202			*Minimal risk of morbidity from additional diagnostic testing or treatment*
99212	*1 self-limited or minor problem*	*Minimal or NONE*	
99221			
99231			
99234			
Low complexity	*2 or more self-limited or minor problems*	*(Must meet 1 of 2 requirements)*	*Low risk of morbidity from additional diagnostic testing or treatment*
99203		**Category 1: Tests and documents**	
99213	*or*	*Any combination of 2 from the following*	
99221	*1 stable, chronic illness*	• *Review of prior external note(s) from each unique source*	
99231	*or*	• *Review of the result(s) of each unique test*	
99234	*1 acute uncomplicated illness or injury*	• *Ordering of each unique test*	
	or	*or*	
	1 stable, acute illness	**Category 2: Assessment requiring an independent historian(s)**	
	or		
	1 acute, uncomplicated illness or injury requiring hospital inpatient or observation level of care		

(Continued)

Example 8.3 (Continued)

MDM (2 out of 3 MDM)	Number of problems	Complexity of data reviewed	Risk of complications and or morbidity
Moderate 99204 99214 99222 99232 99235	1 or more chronic illnesses with exacerbation, progression, or side effects of treatment **or** 2 or more stable chronic illnesses **or** 1 undiagnosed new problem with uncertain prognosis **or** 1 acute illness with systemic symptoms **or** 1 acute, complicated injury	*(Must meet 1 out of 3 requirements)* **Category 1: Tests, documents, historian** *Any combination of 3 from the following* • *Review of prior external note(s) from each unique source** • *Review of the result(s) of each unique test** • *Ordering of each unique test** • *Assessment requiring an independent historian(s)* **or** **Category 2: Independent interpretation of tests** • *Independent interpretation of a test performed by another physician/other qualified healthcare professional (not separately reported)* **or** **Category 3: Discussion of management or test interpretation** • *Discussion of management or test interpretation with external/physician/other qualified healthcare professional/appropriate source (not separately reported)*	*Moderate risk of morbidity from additional diagnostic testing or treatment* Examples only: • *Prescription drug management* • *Decision regarding minor surgery with identified patient or procedure risk factors* • *Decision regarding elective major surgery without identified patient or procedure risk factors* • *Diagnosis or treatment significantly limited by social determinants of health*

High complexity	1 or more chronic illnesses with severe exacerbation, progression, or side effects of treatment	(Must meet 2 out of 3 requirements)	High risk of morbidity from additional diagnostic testing or treatment
99205		**Category 1: Tests, documents, historian**	Examples only:
99215		Any combination of 3 from the following	
99223	**or**	• Review of prior external note(s) from each unique source*	• Drug therapy requiring intensive monitoring for toxicity
99233	1 acute or chronic illness or injury that poses a threat to life or bodily function	• Review of the result(s) of each unique test*	• Decision for elective major surgery with identified patient or procedure risk factors
99236		• Ordering of each unique test*	
		• Assessment requiring an independent historian(s)	

or

Multiple morbidities requiring intensive management (Initial Nursing Facility only)

or

Category 2: Independent interpretation of tests

• Independent interpretation of a test performed by another physician/other qualified healthcare professional (not separately reported)

or

Category 3: Discussion of management or test interpretation

• Discussion of management or test interpretation with external/physician/ other qualified healthcare professional/appropriate source (not separately reported)

• Decision for emergency major surgery

• Decision regarding hospitalization

• Decision for DNR or to de-escalate care because of poor prognosis

• Parenteral controlled substances

Example 9.1 Skilled Nursing Facility services: Subsequent visit

CC	*Follow up on chronic conditions*
HPI	*55-year-old male with pAFib. On Eliquis. Has chronic lymphedema with venous statis ulcers*
Interval development	*Edema has improved greatly with leg wrapping, no open areas noted*
PE	• *Constitution: VS 130/87 P 75 R 16 Weight 182 pounds* • *Resp: CTA bilaterally* • *Cardiac: RRR no murmurs, normal s1s2* • *Ext: bilateral lymphedema with no areas of weeping*
A/P	*1. A fib – continue Eliquis; rate controlled on BB* *2. Lymphedema – continue wound care/leg wrapping* *3. Hypo-albuminemia – protein snacks, recheck CMP in one week*
Provider	*Discussed care with wound care nurse*
Time	*Time spent 20 minutes in review of records, examination of patient, coordination of care, documentation, and placing orders.*

Example 9.2 E/M codes for Nursing Facility Services subsequent visits

E/M code	History/Exam	MDM	Time
99307	*Clinician required to perform and document medically appropriate history and examination*	*Straightforward*	*Or 10 minutes*
99308		*Low*	*Or 15 minutes*
99309		*Moderate*	*Or 30 minutes*
99310		*High*	*Or 45 minutes*

MDM =

Time =

Example 9.3 Medical decision-making tool

MDM (2 out of 3 MDM)	Number of problems	Complexity of data reviewed	Risk of complications and or morbidity
Straightforward 99202 99212 99221 99231 99234	*1 self-limited or minor problem*	*Minimal or NONE*	*Minimal risk of morbidity from additional diagnostic testing or treatment*
Low complexity 99203 99213 99221 99231 99234	*2 or more self-limited or minor problems* **or** *1 stable, chronic illness* **or** *1 acute uncomplicated illness or injury* **or** *1 stable, acute illness* **or** *1 acute, uncomplicated illness or injury requiring hospital inpatient or observation level of care*	*(Must meet 1 of 2 requirements)* **Category 1: Tests and documents** *Any combination of 2 from the following* • *Review of prior external note(s) from each unique source** • *Review of the result(s) of each unique test** • *Ordering of each unique test** **or** **Category 2: Assessment requiring an independent historian(s)**	*Low risk of morbidity from additional diagnostic testing or treatment*

(Continued)

Example 9.3 (Continued)

MDM (2 out of 3 MDM)	Number of problems	Complexity of data reviewed	Risk of complications and or morbidity
Moderate	1 or more chronic illnesses with exacerbation, progression, or side effects of treatment	*(Must meet 1 out of 3 requirements)*	*Moderate risk of morbidity from additional diagnostic testing or treatment*
99204		**Category 1: Tests, documents, historian**	
99214		*Any combination of 3 from the following*	*Examples only:*
99222	**or**	• *Review of prior external note(s) from each unique source**	
99232	2 or more stable chronic illnesses	• *Review of the result(s) of each unique test**	• *Prescription drug management*
99235		• *Ordering of each unique test**	• *Decision regarding minor surgery with identified patient or procedure risk factors*
	or	• *Assessment requiring an independent historian(s)*	
	1 undiagnosed new problem with uncertain prognosis	**or**	• *Decision regarding elective major surgery without identified patient or procedure risk factors*
	or	**Category 2: Independent interpretation of tests**	
	1 acute illness with systemic symptoms	• *Independent interpretation of a test performed by another physician/other qualified healthcare professional (not separately reported)*	• *Diagnosis or treatment significantly limited by social determinants of health*
	or	**or**	
	1 acute, complicated injury	**Category 3: Discussion of management or test interpretation**	
		• *Discussion of management or test interpretation with external/physician/other qualified healthcare professional/appropriate source (not separately reported)*	

High complexity

99205
99215
99223
99233
99236

1 or more chronic illnesses with severe exacerbation, progression, or side effects of treatment

or

1 acute or chronic illness or injury that poses a threat to life or bodily function

or

Multiple morbidities requiring intensive management (Initial Nursing Facility only)

(Must meet 2 out of 3 requirements)

Category 1: Tests, documents, historian

Any combination of 3 from the following

- Review of prior external note(s) from each unique source*
- Review of the result(s) of each unique test*
- Ordering of each unique test*
- Assessment requiring an independent historian(s)

or

Category 2: Independent interpretation of tests

- Independent interpretation of a test performed by another physician/other qualified healthcare professional (not separately reported)

or

Category 3: Discussion of management or test interpretation

- Discussion of management or test interpretation with external/physician/other qualified healthcare professional/appropriate source (not separately reported)

High risk of morbidity from additional diagnostic testing or treatment

Examples only:

- Drug therapy requiring intensive monitoring for toxicity
- Decision for elective major surgery with identified patient or procedure risk factors
- Decision for emergency major surgery
- Decision regarding hospitalization
- Decision for DNR or to de-escalate care because of poor prognosis
- Parenteral controlled substances

DOMICILIARY, REST HOME, OR CUSTODIAL CARE SERVICES

Example 10.1 Domiciliary, rest home, or custodial care services (new patient)

CC	f/u hospital discharge
HPI	55-year-old female recently discharged from hospital 3 days ago with dx of new onset diastolic dysfunction. Weight reported as stable, denies SOB or DOE and states she is able to sleep on 1 pillow.
PFSH	PMH – HTN, HLD CKD stage 3 Fam hx – Mother had breast cancer, Father had COPD
PE	• Constitution: VS 140/98 p 78 R 16 weight 188 (186 on discharge) • Respiratory: CTA no work of breathing • Cardiac: RRR no murmurs – 1+ pedal edema, no JVD • Skin: warm and dry Reviewed labs and Echo from hospital echo shows EF of 55%
A/P	1. New onset diastolic HF – on BB, Lasix, Spiro Aldactone – continue diuretics; check BMP; K at discharge 4.0 2. Unstable HTN – on Ace, diuretic Bp under fair control not at goal of < 140/90 3. HLD – on statin 4. CKD stage 3 – avoid nephrotoxins – reviewed labs GFR 40
TIME	45 minutes spent in review of records, examination of patient, documentation and placing orders

Example 10.2 E/M codes for new patients – domiciliary, rest home, or custodial care services

E/M code	History/Exam	MDM	Time
99341	Clinician required to perform and document medically appropriate history and examination	Straightforward	Or 15 minutes
99342		Low complexity	Or 30 minutes
99344		Mod complexity	Or 60 minutes
99345		High complexity	Or 75 minutes

MDM =

Time =

Example 16.3 Medical decision-making tool

MDM (2 out of 3 MDM)	Number of problems	Complexity of data reviewed	Risk of complications and or morbidity
Straightforward 99202 99212 99221 99231 99234	*1 self-limited or minor problem*	*Minimal or NONE*	*Minimal risk of morbidity from additional diagnostic testing or treatment*
Low complexity 99203 99213 99221 99231 99234	*2 or more self-limited or minor problems* **or** *1 stable, chronic illness* **or** *1 acute uncomplicated illness or injury* **or** *1 stable, acute illness* **or** *1 acute, uncomplicated illness or injury requiring hospital inpatient or observation level of care*	*(Must meet 1 of 2 requirements)* **Category 1: Tests and documents** *Any combination of 2 from the following* • *Review of prior external note(s) from each unique source** • *Review of the result(s) of each unique test** • *Ordering of each unique test** **or** **Category 2: Assessment requiring an independent historian(s)**	*Low risk of morbidity from additional diagnostic testing or treatment*

(Continued)

Example 10.3 (Continued)

MDM (2 out of 3 MDM)	Number of problems	Complexity of data reviewed	Risk of complications and or morbidity
Moderate 99204 99214 99222 99232 99235	1 or more chronic illnesses with exacerbation, progression, or side effects of treatment **or** 2 or more stable chronic illnesses **or** 1 undiagnosed new problem with uncertain prognosis **or** 1 acute illness with systemic symptoms **or** 1 acute, complicated injury	*(Must meet 1 out of 3 requirements)* **Category 1: Tests, documents, historian** *Any combination of 3 from the following* • *Review of prior external note(s) from each unique source** • *Review of the result(s) of each unique test** • *Ordering of each unique test** • *Assessment requiring an independent historian(s)* **or** **Category 2: Independent interpretation of tests** • *Independent interpretation of a test performed by another physician/other qualified healthcare professional (not separately reported)* **or** **Category 3: Discussion of management or test interpretation** • *Discussion of management or test interpretation with external/physician/other qualified healthcare professional/appropriate source (not separately reported)*	*Moderate risk of morbidity from additional diagnostic testing or treatment* Examples only: • *Prescription drug management* • *Decision regarding minor surgery with identified patient or procedure risk factors* • *Decision regarding elective major surgery without identified patient or procedure risk factors* • *Diagnosis or treatment significantly limited by social determinants of health*

High complexity

99205
99215
99223
99233
99236

1 or more chronic illnesses with severe exacerbation, progression, or side effects of treatment

or

1 acute or chronic illness or injury that poses a threat to life or bodily function

or

Multiple morbidities requiring intensive management (Initial Nursing Facility only)

(Must meet 2 out of 3 requirements)

Category 1: Tests, documents, historian

Any combination of 3 from the following

- *Review of prior external note(s) from each unique source**
- *Review of the result(s) of each unique test**
- *Ordering of each unique test**
- *Assessment requiring an independent historian(s)*

or

Category 2: Independent interpretation of tests

- *Independent interpretation of a test performed by another physician/other qualified healthcare professional (not separately reported)*

or

Category 3: Discussion of management or test interpretation

- *Discussion of management or test interpretation with external/physician/ other qualified healthcare professional/appropriate source (not separately reported)*

High risk of morbidity from additional diagnostic testing or treatment

Examples only:

- *Drug therapy requiring intensive monitoring for toxicity*
- *Decision for elective major surgery with identified patient or procedure risk factors*
- *Decision for emergency major surgery*
- *Decision regarding hospitalization*
- *Decision for DNR or to de-escalate care because of poor prognosis*
- *Parenteral controlled substances*

PRACTICE ANSWERS

Example 1.1 New patient office visit

CC   *Establish care*

HPI   *76-year-old female with c/o abdominal pain x 1 week in RUQ –
seems to occur after eating a fatty meal. Pt states attacks are
painful and rates pain 7 out of 10. Nothing seems to make them
better just avoiding certain foods.*

PFSH *Obesity, HTN, HLD*

ROS
- *Constitution: denies weight gain or loss*
- *Resp: denies SOB*
- *Cardiac: denies chest pain/palpitations/syncope*
- *Abdominal: c/o urgent diarrhea after meals at times*

PE
- *Constitutional: VS 130/80 p 99 r 16, appears well*
- *HR: regular heartbeat noted, no edema*
- *Respiration: CTA with normal respiratory effort*
- *GI: RUQ tenderness with positive Murphy's sign*

A/P   *Possible cholecystitis – ordered RUQ ultrasound, CBC, CMP
Referral to surgeon
HTN stable at goal of < 140/80 continue same meds
HLD Lipids reviewed from previous practice and are at goal of < 100;
continue statin*

TIME *45 minutes (review of records, examination of patient, completing
documentation and placing orders)*

DOI: 10.4324/9781003542872-11

Example 1.2 New patient office visit

E/M code	History/Exam	MDM	Time
99202	*Clinician required to perform and document medically appropriate history and examination*	*Straightforward*	*Or 15–29*
99203		*Low complexity*	*Or 30–44*
99204		*Mod complexity*	*Or 45–59*
99205		*High complexity*	*Or 60–74*

MDM = 99204 Moderate

Time = 99204 Moderate

Example 10.3 Medical decision-making tool

MDM (2 out of 3 MDM)	Number of problems	Complexity of data reviewed	Risk of complications and or morbidity
Straightforward 99202 99212 99221 99231 99234	*1 self-limited or minor problem*	*Minimal or NONE*	*Minimal risk of morbidity from additional diagnostic testing or treatment*
Low complexity 99203 99213 99221 99231 99234	*2 or more self-limited or minor problems* **or** *1 stable, chronic illness* **or** *1 acute uncomplicated illness or injury* **or** *1 stable, acute illness* **or** *1 acute, uncomplicated illness or injury requiring hospital inpatient or observation level of care*	*(Must meet 1 of 2 requirements)* **Category 1: Tests and documents** *Any combination of 2 from the following* • *Review of prior external note(s) from each unique source* • *Review of the result (s) of each unique test* • *Ordering of each unique test* *or* **Category 2: Assessment requiring an independent historian(s)**	*Low risk of morbidity from additional diagnostic testing or treatment*

Moderate	(Must meet 1 out of 3 requirements)	*Moderate risk of morbidity from additional diagnostic testing or treatment*
99204	1 or more chronic illnesses with exacerbation, progression, or side effects of treatment	
99214		
99222		Examples only:
99232	**or**	
99235	2 or more stable chronic illnesses	• *Prescription drug management*
	or	• Decision regarding minor surgery with identified patient or procedure risk factors
	1 undiagnosed new problem with uncertain prognosis	
	or	• *Decision regarding elective major surgery without identified patient or procedure risk factors*
	1 acute illness with systemic symptoms	
	or	• Diagnosis or treatment significantly limited by social determinants of health
	1 acute, complicated injury	

Category 1: Tests, documents, historian

Any combination of 3 from the following

• Review of prior external note(s) from each unique source

• *Review of the result(s) of each unique test*

• *Ordering of each unique test*

• Assessment requiring an independent historian(s)

or

Category 2: Independent interpretation of tests

• Independent interpretation of a test performed by another physician/other qualified healthcare professional (not separately reported).

or

Category 3: Discussion of management or test interpretation

• Discussion of management or test interpretation with external/physician/other qualified healthcare professional/appropriate source (not separately reported)

(Continued)

Example 10.3 (Continued)

MDM (2 out of 3 MDM)	Number of problems	Complexity of data reviewed	Risk of complications and or morbidity

High complexity
99205
99215
99223
99233
99236
	1 or more chronic illnesses with severe exacerbation, progression, or side effects of treatment,
	
	or
	
	1 acute or chronic illness or injury that poses a threat to life or bodily function
	
	or
	
	Multiple morbidities requiring intensive management (Initial Nursing Facility only)
		(Must meet 2 out of 3 requirements)
		Category 1: Tests, documents, historian
		Any combination of 3 from the following
		
		  • *Review of prior external note(s) from each unique source*
		  • *Review of the result(s) of each unique test*
		  • *Ordering of each unique test*
		  • *Assessment requiring an independent historian(s)*
		
		or
		
		Category 2: Independent interpretation of tests
		  • *Independent interpretation of a test performed by another physician/other qualified healthcare professional (not separately reported).*
		
		or
		
		Category 3: Discussion of management or test interpretation
		  • *Discussion of management or test interpretation with external/physician/other qualified healthcare professional/appropriate source (not separately reported)*
			High risk of morbidity from additional diagnostic testing or treatment
			Examples only:
			
			  • *Drug therapy requiring intensive monitoring for toxicity*
			  • *Decision for elective major surgery with identified patient or procedure risk factors*
			  • *Decision for emergency major surgery*
			  • *Decision regarding hospitalization*
			  • *Decision for DNR or to de-escalate care because of poor prognosis*
			  • *Parenteral controlled substances*

Example 2.1 Established patient office visit

CC	*c/o left knee pain*
HPI	*12-year-old playing basketball at school reports acute pain in left knee after abrupt turn. States it hurts to bear weight. Rates pain as 10 out of 10. Went to urgent care and they did a CT scan and gave him ibuprofen for the pain*
PFSH	
ROS	
PE	*Constitutional: VS 130/90 p 88 R 16 Weight 98 pounds* *Cardiac: RRR no murmurs* *Skin: Warm and dry* *Extremity: left knee with effusion; Apley maneuver positive, difficult to bear weight.* *CT scan shows meniscal tear (reviewed from Urgent Care)*
A/P	*1. Left knee meniscus tear: knee brace, pain rx, refer to ortho (spoke with orthopedist) school note given for no GYM*
TIME	*45 minutes (review of records, examination of patient, discussion with mother, documentation, discussion with ortho and review of CT scan results, referral to ortho and preparation of discharge paperwork to include prescription)*

Example 2.2 E/M codes for established patient office visit

E/M Code	History /Exam	MDM	Time
99211	*Clinician required to perform and document medically appropriate history and examination*	None	NA
99212		Straightforward	Or 10-19
99213		Low complexity	Or 20-29
99214		Mod complexity	Or 30-39
99215		High complexity	Or 40-54

MDM = 99214 Moderate

Time = 99215 High

Example 2.3 Medical decision-making tool

MDM (2 out of 3 MDM)	Number of problems	Complexity of data reviewed	Risk of complications and or morbidity
Straightforward 99202 99212 99221 99231 99234	*1 self-limited or minor problem*	*Minimal or NONE*	*Minimal risk of morbidity from additional diagnostic testing or treatment*
Low complexity 99203 99213 99221 99231 99234	*2 or more self-limited or minor problems* *or* *1 stable, chronic illness* *or* *1 acute uncomplicated illness or injury* *or* *1 stable, acute illness* *or* *1 acute, uncomplicated illness or injury requiring hospital inpatient or observation level of care*	*(Must meet 1 of 2 requirements of)* **Category 1: Tests and documents** *Any combination of 2 from the following* • *Review of prior external note(s) from each unique source* • *Review of the result(s) of each unique test* • *Ordering of each unique test* *or* **Category 2: Assessment requiring an independent historian(s)**	*Low risk of morbidity from additional diagnostic testing or treatment*

Moderate

99204
99214
99222
99232
99235

1 or more chronic illnesses with exacerbation, progression, or side effects of treatment

or

2 or more stable chronic illnesses

or

1 undiagnosed new problem with uncertain prognosis

or

1 acute illness with systemic symptoms

or

1 acute, complicated injury

(Must meet 1 out of 3 requirements of)

Category 1: Tests, documents, historian

Any combination of 3 from the following

- Review of prior external note(s) from each unique source
- Review of the result(s) of each unique test
- Ordering of each unique test
- Assessment requiring an independent historian(s)

or

Category 2: Independent interpretation of tests

- Independent interpretation of a test performed by another physician/other qualified healthcare professional (not separately reported)

or

Category 3: Discussion of management or test interpretation

- Discussion of management or test interpretation with external/physician/other qualified healthcare professional/appropriate source (not separately reported)

Moderate risk of morbidity from additional diagnostic testing or treatment

Examples only:

- Prescription drug-management
- Decision regarding minor surgery with identified patient or procedure risk factors
- Decision regarding elective major surgery without identified patient or procedure risk factors
- Diagnosis or treatment significantly limited by social determinants of health

(Continued)

Example 2.3 (Continued)

MDM (2 out of 3 MDM)	Number of problems	Complexity of data reviewed	Risk of complications and or morbidity
High complexity 99205 99215 99223 99233 99236	*1 or more chronic illnesses with severe exacerbation, progression, or side effects of treatment* **or** *1 acute or chronic illness or injury that poses a threat to life or bodily function* **or** *Multiple morbidities requiring intensive management (Initial Nursing Facility only)*	*(Must meet 2 out of 3 requirements of)* **Category 1: Tests, documents, historian** *Any combination of 3 from the following* • *Review of prior external note(s) from each unique source* • *Review of the result(s) of each unique test* • *Ordering of each unique test* • *Assessment requiring an independent historian(s)* **or** **Category 2: Independent interpretation of tests** • *Independent interpretation of a test performed by another physician/other qualified healthcare professional (not separately reported)* **or** **Category 3: Discussion of management or test interpretation** • *Discussion of management or test interpretation with external/physician/ other qualified healthcare professional/appropriate*	*High risk of morbidity from additional diagnostic testing or treatment* Examples only: • *Drug therapy requiring intensive monitoring for toxicity* • *Decision for elective major surgery with identified patient or procedure risk factors* • *Decision for emergency major surgery* • *Decision regarding hospitalization* • *Decision for DNR or to de-escalate care because of poor prognosis* • *Parenteral controlled substances*

ACUTE CARE

Example 3.1 Inpatient or initial observation

CC	SOB
HPI	65 yo female with c/o increasing SOB over past 2 days. Pt normally does not wear oxygen now requiring 4 L per nasal cannula. c/o weight gain of 10 pounds over past 3 days with ankle swelling. States she now must sleep on 3 pillows and cannot walk across her living room without resting.
PFSH	PMH HTN Soc hx smokes 1 ppd for past 50 years
ROS	Constitution: c/o weight gain of 10 pounds in last 3 days Lungs: c/o increased SOB with orthopnea Cardiac: denies any chest pressure or palpitations, states her ankles have been swollen
PE	VS 180/80 p 88 r 20 Constitution: alert in minimal distress Resp: obvious WOB cannot complete sentences, Lungs with bilateral rales Cardiac: RRR no murmurs, 2 + pedal edema
DIFF	CHF exacerbation, Pulmonary embolism, Pneumonia
Provider	Spoke with ER physician to admit; spoke with cardiology
A/P	1. New onset Systolic decompensated CHF – reviewed CXR which was normal – pro BNP was 35,000 up from 17,000 last admit 6 months ago; reviewed Echo done 6 months ago by cardiologist, and she had a normal EF of 75% at that time; will start Lasix 40 mg IV BID, monitor daily BMP, consult cardiology, admit to telemetry, and repeat Echo 2. HTN urgency – as evidenced by elevated BP 1870/80 and CKD with GFR of 35 – resume home meds and add hydralazine 50mg TID
TIME	40 minutes (review of records, examination of patient, coordination of care and documentation including orders)

Example 3.2 Initial observation and inpatient E/M codes

E/M code	History/ Exam	MDM	Time
99221	Clinician required to perform and document medically appropriate history and examination	Straightforward or low	Or 40 minutes
99222		Moderate	Or 55 minutes
99223		High	Or 75 minutes

MDM = 99223 High

Time = 99221 Straightforward or low

MDM (2 out of 3 MDM)	Number of problems	Complexity of data reviewed	Risk of complications and or morbidity
Straightforward 99202 99212 99221 99231 99234	*1 self-limited or minor problem*	*Minimal or NONE*	*Minimal risk of morbidity from additional diagnostic testing or treatment*

Low complexity
99203
99213
99221
99231
99234
	2 or more self-limited or minor problems
	
	or
	
	1 stable, chronic illness
	
	or
	
	1 acute uncomplicated illness or injury
	
	or
	
	1 stable, acute illness
	
	or
	
	1 acute, uncomplicated illness or injury requiring hospital inpatient or observation level of care
		(Must meet 1 of 2 requirements)
		Category 1: Tests and documents
		Any combination of 2 from the following
		  • *Review of prior external note(s) from each unique source*
		  • *Review of the result(s) of each unique test*
		  • *Ordering of each unique test*
		
		or
		
		Category 2: Assessment requiring an independent historian(s)
			Low risk of morbidity from additional diagnostic testing or treatment

(Continued)

Example 3.3 (Continued)

MDM (2 out of 3 MDM)	Number of problems	Complexity of data reviewed	Risk of complications and or morbidity
Moderate 99204 99214 99222 99232 99235	1 or more chronic illnesses with exacerbation, progression, or side effects of treatment **or** 2 or more stable chronic illnesses **or** 1 undiagnosed new problem with uncertain prognosis **or** 1 acute illness with systemic symptoms **or** 1 acute, complicated injury **or**	*(Must meet 1 out of 3 requirements of)* **Category 1: Tests, documents, historian** *Any combination of 3 from the following* • *Review of prior external note(s) from each unique source* • *Review of the result(s) of each unique test* • *Ordering of each unique test* • *Assessment requiring an independent historian(s)* **or** **Category 2: Independent interpretation of tests** • *Independent interpretation of a test performed by another physician/other qualified healthcare professional (not separately reported)* **Category 3: Discussion of management or test interpretation** • *Discussion of management or test interpretation with external/physician/other qualified healthcare professional/appropriate source (not separately reported)*	*Moderate risk of morbidity from additional diagnostic testing or treatment* Examples only: • *Prescription drug management* • *Decision regarding minor surgery with identified patient or procedure risk factors* • *Decision regarding elective major surgery without identified patient or procedure risk factors* • *Diagnosis or treatment significantly limited by social determinants of health*

High complexity	1 or more chronic illnesses with severe exacerbation, progression, or side effects of treatment	(Must meet 2 out of 3 requirements of)	High risk of morbidity from additional diagnostic testing or treatment
99205		**Category 1: Tests, documents, historian**	Examples only:
99215		Any combination of 3 from the following	• Drug therapy requiring intensive monitoring for toxicity (Lasix)
99223	**or**	• Review of prior external note(s) from each unique source	• Decision for elective major surgery with identified patient or procedure risk factors
99233	1 acute or chronic illness or injury that poses a threat to life or bodily function	• Review of the result(s) of each unique test	
99236		• Ordering of each unique test	• Decision for emergency major surgery
		• Assessment requiring an independent historian(s)	• Decision regarding hospitalization
	or	**or**	• Decision for DNR or to de-escalate care because of poor prognosis
	Multiple morbidities requiring intensive management (Initial Nursing Facility only)	**Category 2: Independent interpretation of tests**	• Parenteral controlled substances
		• Independent interpretation of a test performed by another physician/other qualified healthcare professional (not separately reported)	
		or	
		Category 3: Discussion of management or test interpretation	
		• Discussion of management or test interpretation with external/physician/other qualified healthcare professional/appropriate	

Example 4.1 Subsequent hospital inpatient and observation services (progress note)

CC	**Back pain**
HPI	*73 yo female pt was admitted for acute back pain x 3 days after coughing fit. Xray shows compression fracture at L3/4. Rates pain 7 out of 10, unable to walk without severe pain*
Interval change	*Vertebroplasty performed; rates pain as 3 out of 10*
PE	*Constitutional — alert x3, appears well* *Muscular skeletal — unsteady gait, walking slowly, normal muscle strength and tone* *Neurological — DTR in lower extremities normal, normal sensation*
Provider	*Ortho has seen patient and has no further interventions planned*
A/P	*1. Compression fracture: PT/OT recommending SNF for rehab — walked 20 feet with walker and SBA, requiring pain rx, start volteran cream TID*
TIME	*20 minutes (review of records, examination of patient, coordination of care and documentation including orders)*

Example 4.2 Subsequent observation and inpatient service E/M codes

E/M code	History/Exam	MDM	Time
99231	*Clinician required to perform and document medically appropriate history and examination*	Straightforward or low	Or 25 minutes
99232		Moderate	Or 35 minutes
99233		High	Or 50 minutes

MDM = 99231 Straightforward or low

Time = does not meet minimum time requirement

MDM (2 out of 3 MDM)	Number of problems	Complexity of data reviewed	Risk of complications and or morbidity
Straight forward 99202 99212 99221 99231 99234	*1 self-limited or minor problem*	*Minimal or NONE*	*Minimal risk of morbidity from additional diagnostic testing or treatment*
Low complexity 99203 99213 99221 99231 99234	*2 or more self-limited or minor problems* **or** *1 stable, chronic illness* **or** *1 acute uncomplicated illness or injury* **or** *1 stable, acute illness* **or** *1 acute, uncomplicated illness or injury requiring hospital inpatient or observation level of care*	*(Must meet 1 of 2 requirements)* **Category 1: Tests and documents** *Any combination of 2 from the following* • *Review of prior external note(s) from each unique source* • *Review of the result(s) of each unique test* • *Ordering of each unique test* *or* **Category 2: Assessment requiring an independent historian(s)**	*Low risk of morbidity from additional diagnostic testing or treatment*

(Continued)

Example 4-3 (Continued)

MDM (2 out of 3 MDM)	Number of problems	Complexity of data reviewed	Risk of complications and or morbidity
Moderate 99204 99214 99222 99232 99235	1 or more chronic illnesses with exacerbation, progression, or side effects of treatment **or** 2 or more stable chronic illnesses. **or** 1 undiagnosed new problem with uncertain prognosis **or** 1 acute illness with systemic symptoms **or** 1 acute, complicated injury	*(Must meet 1 out of 3 requirements)* **Category 1: Tests, documents, historian** *Any combination of 3 from the following* • *Review of prior external note(s) from each unique source* • *Review of the result(s) of each unique test* • *Ordering of each unique test* • *Assessment requiring an independent historian(s)* **or** **Category 2: Independent interpretation of tests** • *Independent interpretation of a test performed by another physician/other qualified healthcare professional (not separately reported)* **or** **Category 3: Discussion of management or test interpretation** • *Discussion of management or test interpretation with external/physician/other qualified healthcare professional/appropriate source (not separately reported)*	*Moderate risk of morbidity from additional diagnostic testing or treatment* Examples only: • *Prescription drug management* • *Decision regarding minor surgery With identified patient or procedure risk factors* • *Decision regarding elective major surgery without identified patient or procedure risk factors* • *Diagnosis or treatment significantly limited by social determinants of health*

High complexity

99205
99215
99223
99233
99236

1 or more chronic illnesses with severe exacerbation, progression, or side effects of treatment

or

1 acute or chronic illness or injury that poses a threat to life or bodily function

or

Multiple morbidities requiring intensive management (Initial Nursing Facility only)

(Must meet 2 out of 3 requirements)

Category 1: Tests, documents, historian

Any combination of 3 from the following

- *Review of prior external note(s) from each unique source*
- *Review of the result(s) of each unique test*
- *Ordering of each unique test*
- *Assessment requiring an independent historian(s)*

or

Category 2: Independent interpretation of tests

- *Independent interpretation of a test performed by another physician/other qualified healthcare professional (not separately reported)*

or

Category 3: Discussion of management or test interpretation

- *Discussion of management or test interpretation with external/physician/other qualified healthcare professional/appropriate*

High risk of morbidity from additional diagnostic testing or treatment

Examples only:

- *Drug therapy requiring intensive monitoring for toxicity*
- *Decision for elective major surgery with identified patient or procedure risk factors*
- *Decision for emergency major surgery*
- *Decision regarding hospitalization*
- *Decision for DNR or to de-escalate care because of poor prognosis*
- *Parenteral controlled substances*

Example 5.1 Admit/discharge same day

CC	*Abdominal pain*
HPI	*17 yo female with 1 day h/o epigastric abdominal pain that has been increasing. Pt states it is knifelike. Rates severity 8 out of 10. Movement makes it worse; nothing seems to make it better.*
PFSH	*No sig PMH*
ROS	*C/o feeling feverish; c/o RLQ abdominal pain as per HPI* *c/o nausea*
PE	*VS 100/80 76 16, appears unwell* *ENT: nares patent with no drainage, no posterior pharynx erythema* *Resp: CTA bilaterally- normal respiratory effort* *Cardiac: RRR-, no pedal edema* *Abd: guarded with positive McBurney, positive heel-jar* *Skin: warm and dry* *CT of abdomen shows acute appendicitis* *WBC count 18,000*
DIFF	*Acute appendicitis; Pelvic inflammatory disease; acute gallbladder disease; ectopic pregnancy, ovarian cyst*
Provider	*Accepted patient from ER; Spoke with surgeon after procedure ; Reviewed all lab work*
Admission Dx	*Acute Appendicitis*
Discharge Dx	*Acute Appendicitis s/p lab appendectomy*
Dispo	*HOME*
Code status	*FULL*
Condition	*GOOD*
Discharge instructions	*No heavy lifting x 1 week, no tub baths for 1 week; PRN Percocet given for pain; as well as Colace 100mg BID*
TIME	*65 minutes*

Example 5.2 Admit/DC same day observation and inpatient E/M codes

E/M code	History/Exam	MDM	Time
99234-	Clinician required to perform and document medically appropriate history and examination	Straightforward or Low	Or 40 minutes
99235-		Moderate	Or 70 minutes
99236-		High	Or 85 minutes

MDM = 99235 Moderate

Time = 99234

Example 5.3 Medical decision-making tool

MDM (2 out of 3 MDM)	Number of problems	Complexity of data reviewed	Risk of complications and or morbidity
Straightforward 99202 99212 99221 99231 99234	*1 self-limited or minor problem*	*Minimal or NONE*	*Minimal risk of morbidity from additional diagnostic testing or treatment*
Low complexity 99203 99213 99221 99231 99234	*2 or more self-limited or minor problems* **or** *1 stable, chronic illness* **or** *1 acute uncomplicated illness or injury* **or** *1 stable, acute illness* **or** *1 acute, uncomplicated illness or injury requiring hospital inpatient or observation level of care*	*(Must meet 1 of 2 requirements)* **Category 1: Tests and documents** *Any combination of 2 from the following* • *Review of prior external note(s) from each unique source* • *Review of the result(s) of each unique test* • *Ordering of each unique test* **or** **Category 2: Assessment requiring an independent historian(s)**	*Low risk of morbidity from additional diagnostic testing or treatment*

Moderate	(Must meet 1 out of 3 requirements)	*Moderate risk of morbidity from additional diagnostic testing or treatment*
99204	1 or more chronic illnesses with exacerbation, progression, or side effects of treatment	
99214		
99222		Examples only:
99232		
99235		

1 or more chronic illnesses with exacerbation, progression, or side effects of treatment

or

2 or more stable chronic illnesses

or

1 undiagnosed new problem with uncertain prognosis

or

1 acute illness with systemic symptoms

or

1 acute, complicated injury

Moderate risk of morbidity from additional diagnostic testing or treatment

Examples only:

- *Prescription drug-management*
- *Decision regarding minor surgery with identified patient or procedure risk factors*
- *Decision regarding elective major surgery without identified patient or procedure risk factors*
- *Diagnosis or treatment significantly limited by social determinants of health*

Category 1: Tests, documents, historian

Any combination of 3 from the following

- *Review of prior external note(s) from each unique source*
- *Review of the result(s) of each unique test*
- *Ordering of each unique test*
- *Assessment requiring an independent historian(s)*

or

Category 2: Independent interpretation of tests

- *Independent interpretation of a test performed by another physician/other qualified healthcare professional (not separately reported)*

or

Category 3: Discussion of management or test interpretation

- *Discussion of management or test interpretation with external/physician/other qualified healthcare professional/appropriate source (not separately reported)*

(Continued)

Example 5-3 (Continued)

MDM (2 out of 3 MDM)	Number of problems	Complexity of data reviewed	Risk of complications and or morbidity
High complexity 99205 99215 99223 99233 99236	*1 or more chronic illnesses with severe exacerbation, progression, or side effects of treatment* **or** *1 acute or chronic illness or injury that poses a threat to life or bodily function* **or** *Multiple morbidities requiring intensive management (Initial Nursing Facility only)*	*(Must meet 2 out of 3 requirements)* **Category 1: Tests, documents, historian** *Any combination of 3 from the following* • *Review of prior external note(s) from each unique source* • *Review of the result(s) of each unique test* • *Ordering of each unique test* • *Assessment requiring an independent historian(s)* **or** **Category 2: Independent interpretation of tests** • *Independent interpretation of a test performed by another physician/other qualified healthcare professional (not separately reported)* **or** **Category 3: Discussion of management or test interpretation** • *Discussion of management or test interpretation with external/physician/other qualified healthcare professional/appropriate*	*High risk of morbidity from additional diagnostic testing or treatment* Examples only: • *Drug therapy requiring intensive monitoring for toxicity* • *Decision for elective major surgery with identified patient or procedure risk factors* • *Decision for emergency major surgery* • *Decision regarding hospitalization* • *Decision for DNR or to de-escalate care because of poor prognosis* • *Parenteral controlled substances*

HOSPITAL DISCHARGE

Example 6.1 Hospital discharge note

Day of admission	*5/2/2022*
Day of discharge	*5/4/2022*
Discharge diagnosis	*Chest pain – noncardiac* *Muscle strain*
Brief physical exam	• *Alert x 3* • *Cardiac – RRR* • *Resp – CTA* • *Skin – warm and dry*
Hospital course	*48-year-old male admitted with c/o exertional chest pain. Rated pain a 7 out of 10. Cardiac markers x 3 neg, EKG normal. Stress test did not show signs of ischemia. Pt pain improved with Toradol. Normal kidney function.*
Discharge meds	*None; may take OTC Motrin or Aleve for pain, use diclofenac cream QID*
Additional tests	*No further tests needed*
Follow up	*f/u with Primary care doctor in 7 days*
Dispo	*Home*
Condition	*Good*
Code	*Full*
Time	*Total time spent in review of record, physical exam, coordination of care with care givers and preparation of discharge paperwork is 35 minutes*

Example 6.2 Hospital discharge day management E/M coding

E/M code	Face-to-face encounter	Time
99238	*Clinician required to perform and document medically appropriate history and examination*	≤ 30 minutes
99239		≥ 30 minutes

Time = 99239

Example 7.1 Emergency room

CC	*Complaint of left ear pain*
HPI	*8-month-old infant with c/o pulling on left ear, crying when laid down, fever x1 day. Max temp in last 24 hours 102.6 under arm, improved with Aleve reported per mother*
PFSH	*No significant PMH; parents do smoke in the house*
ROS	• *Constitution: mother reports max temp 102.6* • *ENT: Mother reports pulling on left ear, mother reports some clear nasal drainage* • *GI: Mother denies decreased appetite, vomiting or diarrhea*
PE	• *Constitution: T 103 P 90 R 16, fussy* • *ENT: Left TM bulging with fluid in middle ear, nares with clear drainage, posterior pharynx red with petechial rash on pillars* • *Resp: CTA bilaterally* • *Skin: warm, dry, no rash*
DIFF	*Otitis Media; Serous Otitis Media; Viral Pharyngitis; Strep Pharyngitis*
Provider	*NA*
Testing	**Strep test positive**
Dx	1. *Strep throat – per rapid test – prescribed amoxicillin* 2. *Left acute OM – on higher dose of amoxicillin for 10 days*
Discharge instructions	*Complete all antibiotics; return to PCP or clinic if no improvement in next 24 hours*
TIME	*24 minutes*

Example 7.2 Emergency room E/M coding

E/M code	History/Exam	MDM
99281	*Clinician required to perform and document medically appropriate history and examination*	*N/A*
99282		*Straightforward*
99283-		*Low*
99284		*Moderate*
99285		*High*

MDM = 99283 Low

NO TIME COMPONENT (Note you could add a 25 modifier and ADD on preventive counseling code based on the time you spent for smoking cessation and increased ear infections in children.)

Example 7.3 Medical decision-making tool

MDM (2 out of 3 MDM)	Number of problems	Complexity of data reviewed	Risk of complications and or morbidity
Straightforward 99202 99212 99221 99231 99234	1 self-limited or minor problem	Minimal or NONE	Minimal risk of morbidity from additional diagnostic testing or treatment
Low complexity 99203 99213 99221 99231 99234	2 or more self-limited or minor problems, or 1 stable, chronic illness, or 1 acute uncomplicated illness or injury or 1 stable, acute illness or 1 acute, uncomplicated illness or injury requiring hospital inpatient or observation level of care	(Must meet 1 of 2 requirements) **Category 1: Tests and documents** Any combination of 2 from the following • Review of prior external note(s) from each unique source • Review of the result(s) of each unique test • Ordering of each unique test or **Category 2: Assessment requiring an independent historian(s)**	Low risk of morbidity from additional diagnostic testing or treatment

Moderate	1 or more chronic illnesses with exacerbation, progression, or side effects of treatment	(Must meet 1 out of 3 requirements)	Moderate risk of morbidity from additional diagnostic testing or treatment
99204		**Category 1: Tests, documents, historian**	
99214		Any combination of 3 from the following	Examples only:
99222	or	• Review of prior external note(s) from each unique source	• *Prescription drug management*
99232	2 or more stable chronic illnesses	• Review of the result(s) of each unique test	• Decision regarding minor surgery with identified patient or procedure risk factors
99235	or	• Ordering of each unique test	• Decision regarding elective major surgery without identified patient or procedure risk factors
	1 undiagnosed new problem with uncertain prognosis	• Assessment requiring an independent historian(s)	• Diagnosis or treatment significantly limited by social determinants of health
	or	or	
	1 acute illness with systemic symptoms	**Category 2: Independent interpretation of tests**	
		• Independent interpretation of a test performed by another physician/other qualified healthcare professional (not separately reported)	
	or	or	
	1 acute, complicated injury	**Category 3: Discussion of management or test interpretation**	
		• Discussion of management or test interpretation with external/physician/other qualified healthcare professional/appropriate source (not separately reported)	

(Continued)

Example 7.3 (Continued)

MDM (2 out of 3 MDM)	Number of problems	Complexity of data reviewed	Risk of complications and or morbidity
High complexity 99205 99215 99223 99233 99236	*1 or more chronic illnesses with severe exacerbation, progression, or side effects of treatment* **or** *1 acute or chronic illness or injury that poses a threat to life or bodily function* **or** *Multiple morbidities requiring intensive management (Initial Nursing Facility only)*	*(Must meet 2 out of 3 requirements)* **Category 1: Tests, documents, historian** *Any combination of 3 from the following* • *Review of prior external note(s) from each unique source* • *Review of the result(s) of each unique test* • *Ordering of each unique test* • *Assessment requiring an independent historian(s)* **or** **Category 2: Independent interpretation of tests** • *Independent interpretation of a test performed by another physician/other qualified healthcare professional (not separately reported)* **or** **Category 3: Discussion of management or test interpretation** • *Discussion of management or test interpretation with external/physician/other qualified healthcare professional/appropriate source (not separately reported)*	*High risk of morbidity from additional diagnostic testing or treatment* Examples only: • *Drug therapy requiring intensive monitoring for toxicity* • *Decision for elective major surgery with identified patient or procedure risk factors* • *Decision for emergency major surgery* • *Decision regarding hospitalization* • *Decision for DNR or to de-escalate care because of poor prognosis* • *Parenteral controlled substances*

SKILLED NURSING FACILITY SERVICES

Example 8.1 Skilled Nursing Facility Services: Initial visit

CC *Failing to thrive*

HPI *86-year-old female with failure to thrive. Comes from hospital with decreased appetite and loss of 20 pounds past several months, w/u did not reveal underlying cause. Spoke to daughter about previous level of function prior to Covid 19*

PFSH *PMH HTN, HLD, DM type 2, Depression, Macular degeneration, Covid 19 3 months ago*
Fam hx — parents deceased
Soc hx — denies smoking, ETOH socially

ROS
- *Constitution: c/o fatigue*
- *Resp: denies SOB, DOE, or orthopnea*
- *Cardiac: denies CP or palpitations*
- *GI: c/o no appetite since Covid 19; occasional diarrhea*
- *Psychiatric: c/o lack of interest in activities*

PE
- *Constitution: VS 120/80 P 80 R 20 weight 98 pounds*
- *Respiratory: decreased breath sounds bilaterally*
- *Cardiac: RRR no murmurs, thrills; no edema*
- *Skin: warm and dry without rashes*
- *Psyc: good insight and judgment: PHQ 9 15 (moderate depression)*

A/P *Review and summation of old records*
- *Long Haul Covid — continue nebs*
- *Depression — start Remeron 7.5mg nightly*
- *Severe malnutrition — dietary consult; check albumin*
- *Stable HTN — at goal of < 140/90 continue Lisinopril/ HCTZ*
- *Stable DM type 2 — HgA1c last at goal of < 7 — diabetic diet — continue metformin*
- *Discussed end of life care for 30 minutes with advance directive paperwork on file, decision made to deescalate care and consult hospice*

TIME *Total time spent 55 minutes in review of hospital records, examination of patient, finalization of admission orders to include medication reconciliation, and ordering of lab work.*

Example 8.2 E/M codes for Initial Nursing Facility services

E/M code	History/Exam	MDM	Time
99304	Clinician required to perform and document medically appropriate history and examination	Straightforward or Low	Or 25 minutes
99305		Moderate	Or 35 minutes
99306		High	Or 45 minutes

MDM = 99306 High

Time = 99306

(Note you could add modifier 25 and bill for advance care planning based on the time you spent.)

Example 8.3 Medical decision-making tool

MDM (2 out of 3 MDM)	Number of problems	Complexity of data reviewed	Risk of complications and or morbidity
Straightforward 99202 99212 99221 99231 99234	*1 self-limited or minor problem*	*Minimal or NONE*	*Minimal risk of morbidity from additional diagnostic testing or treatment*
Low complexity 99203 99213 99221 99231 99234	*2 or more self-limited or minor problems* **or** *1 stable, chronic illness* **or** *1 acute uncomplicated illness or injury* **or** *1 stable, acute illness* **or** *1 acute, uncomplicated illness or injury requiring hospital inpatient or observation level of care*	*(Must meet 1 of 2 requirements)* **Category 1: Tests and documents** *Any combination of 2 from the following* • *Review of prior external note(s) from each unique source* • *Review of the result(s) of each unique test* • *Ordering of each unique test* *or* **Category 2: Assessment requiring an independent historian(s)**	*Low risk of morbidity from additional diagnostic testing or treatment*

(Continued)

Example 8.3 (Continued)

MDM (2 out of 3 MDM)	Number of problems	Complexity of data reviewed	Risk of complications and or morbidity
Moderate 99204 99214 99222 99232 99235	1 or more chronic illnesses with exacerbation, progression, or side effects of treatment or 2 or more stable chronic illnesses or 1 undiagnosed new problem with uncertain prognosis or 1 acute illness with systemic symptoms or 1 acute, complicated injury	*(Must meet 1 out of 3 requirements)* **Category 1: Tests, documents, historian** *Any combination of 3 from the following* • *Review of prior external note(s) from each unique source* • *Review of the result(s) of each unique test* • *Ordering of each unique test* • *Assessment requiring an independent historian(s)* or **Category 2: Independent interpretation of tests** • *Independent interpretation of a test performed by another physician/other qualified healthcare professional (not separately reported)* or **Category 3: Discussion of management or test interpretation** • *Discussion of management or test interpretation with external/physician/other qualified healthcare professional/appropriate source (not separately reported)*	*Moderate risk of morbidity from additional diagnostic testing or treatment* Examples only: • *Prescription drug management* • *Decision regarding minor surgery with identified patient or procedure risk factors* • *Decision regarding elective major surgery without identified patient or procedure risk factors* • *Diagnosis or treatment significantly limited by social determinants of health*

| **High complexity**
99205
99215
99223
99233
99236 | 1 or more chronic illnesses with severe exacerbation, progression, or side effects of treatment

or

1 acute or chronic illness or injury that poses a threat to life or bodily function

or

Multiple morbidities requiring intensive management (Initial Nursing Facility only) | (Must meet 2 out of 3 requirements)

Category 1: Tests, documents, historian
Any combination of 3 from the following
• Review of prior external note(s) from each unique source
• Review of the result(s) of each unique test
• Ordering of each unique test
• Assessment requiring an independent historian(s)

or

Category 2: Independent interpretation of tests
• Independent interpretation of a test performed by another physician/other qualified healthcare professional (not separately reported)

or

Category 3: Discussion of management or test interpretation
• Discussion of management or test interpretation with external/physician/ other qualified healthcare professional/appropriate source (not separately reported) | High risk of morbidity from additional diagnostic testing or treatment
Examples only:
• Drug therapy requiring intensive monitoring for toxicity
• Decision for elective major surgery with identified patient or procedure risk factors
• Decision for emergency major surgery
• Decision regarding hospitalization
• Decision for DNR or to de-escalate care because of poor prognosis
• Parenteral controlled substances |

Example 9.1 Skilled Nursing Facility services: Subsequent visit

CC	*Follow up on chronic conditions*
HPI	*55-year-old male with pAFib. On Eliquis. Has chronic lymphedema with venous statis ulcers*
Interval development	*Edema has improved greatly with leg wrapping, no open areas noted*
PE	• *Constitution: VS 130/87 P 75 R 16 Weight 182 pounds* • *Resp: CTA bilaterally* • *Cardiac: RRR no murmurs, normal s1s2* • *Ext: bilateral lymphedema with no areas of weeping*
A/P	*1. A fib – continue Eliquis; rate controlled on beta-blocker (target less than 100)* *2. Lymphedema – continue wound care/leg wrapping –* *3. hypo-albuminemia – protein snacks, recheck CMP in one week*
Provider	*Discussed care with wound care nurse*
TIME	*Time spent 20 minutes in review of records, examination of patient, coordination of care, documentation, and placing orders.*

Example 9.2 E/M codes for Nursing Facility Services subsequent visits

E/M code	History/Exam	MDM	Time
99307		*Straightforward*	*Or 10 minutes*
99308	*Clinician required to perform and document medically appropriate history and examination*	*LOW*	*Or 15 minutes*
99309		*Moderate*	*Or 30 minutes*
99310		*HIGH*	*Or 45 minutes*

MDM = 99309 Moderate

Time = 99308 Low

Example 9.3 Medical decision-making tool

MDM (2 out of 3 MDM)	Number of problems	Complexity of data reviewed	Risk of complications and or morbidity
Straightforward 99202 99212 99221 99231 99234	*1 self-limited or minor problem*	*Minimal or NONE*	*Minimal risk of morbidity from additional diagnostic testing or treatment*
Low complexity 99203 99213 99221 99231 99234	*2 or more self-limited or minor problems* **or** *1 stable, chronic illness* **or** *1 acute uncomplicated illness or injury* **or** *1 stable, acute illness* **or** *1 acute, uncomplicated illness or injury requiring hospital inpatient or observation level of care*	*(Must meet 1 of 2 requirements)* **Category 1: Tests and documents** *Any combination of 2 from the following* • *Review of prior external note(s) from each unique sourc* • *Review of the result(s) of each unique test* • *Ordering of each unique test* *or* **Category 2: Assessment requiring an independent historian(s)**	*Low risk of morbidity from additional diagnostic testing or treatment*

(Continued)

Example 9.3 (Continued)

MDM (2 out of 3 MDM)	Number of problems	Complexity of data reviewed	Risk of complications and or morbidity
Moderate 99204 99214 99222 99232 99235	1 or more chronic illnesses with exacerbation, progression, or side effects of treatment *or* 2 or more stable chronic illnesses *or* 1 undiagnosed new problem with uncertain prognosis *or* 1 acute illness with systemic symptoms *or* 1 acute, complicated injury	*(Must meet 1 out of 3 requirements)* **Category 1: Tests, documents, historian** *Any combination of 3 from the following* • *Review of prior external note(s) from each unique source* • *Review of the result(s) of each unique test* • *Ordering of each unique test* • *Assessment requiring an independent historian(s)* *or* **Category 2: Independent interpretation of tests** • *Independent interpretation of a test performed by another physician/other qualified healthcare professional (not separately reported)* *or* **Category 3: Discussion of management or test interpretation** • *Discussion of management or test interpretation with external/physician/other qualified healthcare professional/appropriate source (not separately reported)*	*Moderate risk of morbidity from additional diagnostic testing or treatment* Examples only: • *Prescription drug management* • *Decision regarding minor surgery with identified patient or procedure risk factors* • *Decision regarding elective major surgery without identified patient or procedure risk factors* • *Diagnosis or treatment significantly limited by social determinants of health*

High complexity	*1 or more chronic illnesses with severe exacerbation, progression, or side effects of treatment*	*(Must meet 2 out of 3 requirements)*	*High risk of morbidity from additional diagnostic testing or treatment*
99205		**Category 1: Tests, documents, historian**	Examples only:
99215	**or**	*Any combination of 3 from the following*	
99223	*1 acute or chronic illness or injury that poses a threat to life or bodily function*	• *Review of prior external note(s) from each unique source*	• *Drug therapy requiring intensive monitoring for toxicity*
99233		• *Review of the result(s) of each unique test*	• *Decision for elective major surgery with identified patient or procedure risk factors*
99236	**or**	• *Ordering of each unique test*	• *Decision for emergency major surgery*
	Multiple morbidities requiring intensive management (Initial Nursing Facility only)	• *Assessment requiring an independent historian(s)*	• *Decision regarding hospitalization*
		or	• *Decision for DNR or to de-escalate care because of poor prognosis*
		Category 2: Independent interpretation of tests	• *Parenteral controlled substances*
		• *Independent interpretation of a test performed by another physician/other qualified healthcare professional (not separately reported)*	
		or	
		Category 3: Discussion of management or test interpretation	
		• *Discussion of management or test interpretation with external/physician/other qualified healthcare professional/appropriate source (not separately reported)*	

DOMICILIARY, REST HOME, OR CUSTODIAL CARE SERVICES

Example 10.1 Domiciliary, rest home, or custodial care services (new patient)

CC   *f/u hospital discharge*

HPI   *55-year-old female recently discharged from hospital 3 days ago with dx of new onset diastolic dysfunction. Weight reported as stable, denies SOB or DOE and states she can now sleep on 1 pillow.*

PFSH   *PMH – HTN, HLD CKD stage 3*
          Fam hx – Mother had breast cancer, Father had COPD

PE   • *Constitution: VS 140/98 (goal is < 140/90) p 78 R 16 weight 188 (186 on discharge) (Goal weight 185)*
          • *Respiratory: CTA no work of breathing*
          • *Cardiac: RRR no murmurs- 1+ pedal edema, no JVD*
          • *Skin: warm and dry*
          Reviewed labs and Echo from hospital Echo shows EF of 55%

A/P   1. *New onset diastolic HF – on BB, Lasix, Spiro Aldactone – increase diuretics; check BMP every week; K at discharge 4.0*
          2. *Unstable HTN – on Ace, diuretic Bp under fair control not at goal of < 140/90 will see what affect increased diuretic have may need to add hydralazine*
          3. *HLD – lipids at goal of < 100 (reviewed previous record) on statin*
          4. *CKD stage 3 – avoid nephrotoxins – reviewed labs GFR 40*

Time *45 minutes spent in review of records, examination of patient, documentation and placing orders*

Example 10.2 E/M codes for new patients – domiciliary, rest home, or custodial care services

E/M code	History/Exam	MDM	Time
99341- NEW	Clinician required to perform and document medically appropriate history and examination	Straightforward	Or 15 minutes
99342- NEW		Low Complexity	Or 30 minutes
99344-NEW		Mod Complexity	Or 60 minutes
99345-NEW		High Complexity	Or 75 minutes

MDM = 99344 Moderate

Time = 99342 Low

(Note on this visit you could also add modifier 25 and add on preventive counseling code based on the time you spent if you talked about a heart healthy diet for CHF.)

Example 10.3 Medical decision-making tool

MDM (2 out of 3 MDM)	Number of problems	Complexity of data reviewed	Risk of complications and or morbidity
Straightforward 99202 99212 99221 99231 99234	*1 self-limited or minor problem*	*Minimal or NONE*	*Minimal risk of morbidity from additional diagnostic testing or treatment*
Low complexity 99203 99213 99221 99231 99234	*2 or more self-limited or minor problems* **or** *1 stable, chronic illness* **or** *1 acute uncomplicated illness or injury* **or** *1 stable, acute illness* **or** *1 acute, uncomplicated illness or injury requiring hospital inpatient or observation level of care*	*(Must meet 1 of 2 requirements of)* **Category 1: Tests and documents** *Any combination of 2 from the following* • *Review of prior external note(s) from each unique source* • *Review of the result(s) of each unique test* • *Ordering of each unique test* *or* **Category 2: Assessment requiring an independent historian(s)**	*Low risk of morbidity from additional diagnostic testing or treatment*

Moderate	(Must meet 1 out of 3 requirements of)	*Moderate risk of morbidity from additional diagnostic testing or treatment*
99204 99214 99222 99232 99235	**Category 1: Tests, documents, historian** Any combination of 3 from the following	Examples only:

1 or more chronic illnesses with exacerbation, progression, or side effects of treatment

or

2 or more stable chronic illnesses

or

1 undiagnosed new problem with uncertain prognosis

or

1 acute illness with systemic symptoms

or

1 acute, complicated injury

Category 1: Tests, documents, historian
Any combination of 3 from the following
- *Review of prior external note(s) from each unique source*
- *Review of the result(s) of each unique test*
- *Ordering of each unique test*
- *Assessment requiring an independent historian(s)*

or

Category 2: Independent interpretation of tests
- *Independent interpretation of a test performed by another physician/other qualified healthcare professional (not separately reported)*

or

Category 3: Discussion of management or test interpretation
- *Discussion of management or test interpretation with external/physician/other qualified healthcare professional/appropriate source (not separately reported)*

Moderate risk of morbidity from additional diagnostic testing or treatment
Examples only:
- *Prescription drug management*
- *Decision regarding minor surgery with identified patient or procedure risk factors*
- *Decision regarding elective major surgery without identified patient or procedure risk factors*
- *Diagnosis or treatment significantly limited by social determinants of health*

(Continued)

Example 10.3 (Continued)

MDM (2 out of 3 MDM)	Number of problems	Complexity of data reviewed	Risk of complications and or morbidity
High complexity 99205 99215 99223 99233 99236	*1 or more chronic illnesses with severe exacerbation, progression, or side effects of treatment,* **or** *1 acute or chronic illness or injury that poses a threat to life or bodily function* **or** *Multiple morbidities requiring intensive management (Initial Nursing Facility only)*	*(Must meet 2 out of 3 requirements)* **Category 1: Tests, documents, historian** *Any combination of 3 from the following* • *Review of prior external note(s) from each unique source* • *Review of the result(s) of each unique test* • *Ordering of each unique test* • *Assessment requiring an independent historian(s)* **or** **Category 2: Independent interpretation of tests** • *Independent interpretation of a test performed by another physician/other qualified healthcare professional (not separately reported)* **or** **Category 3: Discussion of management or test interpretation** • *Discussion of management or test interpretation with external/physician/ other qualified healthcare professional/appropriate source (not separately reported)*	*High risk of morbidity from additional diagnostic testing or treatment* Examples only: • *Drug therapy requiring intensive monitoring for toxicity* • *Decision for elective major surgery with identified patient or procedure risk factors* • *Decision for emergency major surgery* • *Decision regarding hospitalization* • *Decision for DNR or to de-escalate care because of poor prognosis* • *Parenteral controlled substances*

TOOLS AND RESOURCES

- United States Preventive Task Force (screening recommendations)
  https://www.uspreventiveservicestaskforce.org/uspstf/

- CDC vaccines & immunizations
  https://www.cdc.gov/vaccines/index.html

- American Academy of Pediatrics Bright Futures (wellness guidelines)
  https://www.aap.org/en/practice-management/bright-futures

- Substance screening and assessment tools
  https://nida.nih.gov/nidamed-medical-health-professionals/screening-tools-resources/chart-screening-tools

- SLUMS examination (dementia)
  https://www.slu.edu/medicine/internal-medicine/geriatric-medicine/aging-successfully/-pdf/slums-form.pdf

- GET up and Go test
  https://www.cdc.gov/steadi/media/pdfs/STEADI-Assessment-TUG-508.pdf

- PHQ9 (depression screening)
  https://www.mdcalc.com/calc/1725/phq9-patient-health-questionnaire9

DOI: 10.4324/9781003542872-12

- Advance directive forms
  https://www.aarp.org/caregiving/financial-legal/free-printable-advance-directives/?cmp=KNC-DSO-CAREGIVING-AdvanceDirectives-22760-GOOG-AdvancedDirectivesForms-Exact-NonBrand&gclid=EAIaIQobChMItczw-aOd_AIVihXUAR0jcQAgEAAYASAAEgJYg_D_BwE&gclsrc=aw.ds

- Medicare wellness exams
  https://www.medicare.gov/coverage/yearly-wellness-visits

- American Medical Association E/M Code and Guideline Changes
  https://www.ama-assn.org/system/files/2023-e-m-descriptors-guidelines.pdf

Table 12.1 AMA 2022 wRVU for E/M codes with reimbursement

E/M code	Short description	Non-facility price ($)	Facility price ($)	Work RVU
99202	*Office o/p new SF 15–29 min*	72.86	48.12	0.93
99203	*Office o/p new low 30–44 min*	112.84	83.02	1.6
99204	*Office o/p new mod 45–59 min*	167.40	133.52	2.6
99205	*Office o/p new high 60–84 min*	220.95	181.30	3.5
99211	*Office/op established may does NOT require physician or QHP*	23.38	8.81	0.18
99212	*Office o/p est SF 10–19 min*	56.93	35.58	0.7
99213	*Office o/p est low 20–29 min*	90.82	66.08	1.3
99214	*Office o/p est mod 30–39 min*	128.43	97.60	1.92
99215	*Office o/p est high 40–54 min*	179.94	143.34	2.8
99221	*1st hosp IP/obs SF low 40*	83.36	83.36	1.63
99222	*1st hosp IP/obs mod 55 min*	130.47	130.47	2.6
99223	*1st hosp IP/obs high 75*	173.84	173.84	3.5

(Continued)

Table 12.1 (Continued)

E/M code	Short description	Non-facility price ($)	Facility price ($)	Work RVU
99231	Sub hosp IP/obs SF/low 25	49.81	49.81	1
99232	Sbsq hosp IP/obs mod 35	79.30	79.30	1.59
99233	Sbsq hosp IP/obs high 50	119.28	119.28	2.4
99234	Hosp IP/obs same date SF/low 45	98.95	98.95	2
99235	Hosp IP/obs same date mod 70	159.61	159.61	3.24
99236	Hosp IP/obs same date high 85	209.08	209.08	4.3
99238	Hosp IP/obs disc mgmt < 30	80.99	80.99	1.5
99239	Hosp IP/obs disc mgmt >30	114.88	114.88	2.15
99281	EMR dpt vst mayx req phy/qhp	11.86	11.86	0.25
99282	Emergency dept visit SF MDM	42.04	42.02	0.93
99283	Emergency dept visit low MDM	72.18	72.18	1.6
99284	Emergency dept visit mod MDM	121.32	121.32	2.74
99285	Emergency dept visit high MDM	176.55	176.55	4
99291	Critical care first hour	275.50	213.83	4.5
99292	Critical care addl 30 min	120.30	107.42	2.25
99304	1st NF care SF/low MDM 25	80.65	80.65	1.5
99305	1st NF care moderate MDM 35	133.52	133.52	2.5
99306	1st NF care high MDM 45	182.31	182.31	3.5
99307	Sbsq NF care SF MDM 10	39.65	39.65	0.7
99308	Sbsq NF care low MDM 15	74.55	74.55	1.3
99309	Sbsq NF care moderate MDM 30	106.75	106.75	1.92
99310	Sbsq NF care high MDM 45	153.51	153.51	2.8

(Continued)

Table 12.1 (Continued)

E/M code	Short description	Non-facility price ($)	Facility price ($)	Work RVU
99315	NF dschrg mgmt 30 min/less	81.67	81.67	1.5
99316	NF dschrg mgmt 30 min +	131.48	131.48	2.5
99341	Home/res vst newSF MDM 15	48.80	48.80	1
99342	Home/res vst new Low MDM 30	77.94	77.94	1.65
99344	Home/res vst new Mod MDM 60	s144.02	144.02	2.87
99345	Home/res vst new high MDM 75	202.65	202.65	3.88
99347	Home/res vst test SF MDM 20	44.73	44.73	0.9
99348	Home/res vst test low MDM 30	76.25	76.45	1.5
99349	Home/res vst test mod MDM 40	127.76	127.76	2.44
99350	Home/res vst test high MDM 75	202.65	202.65	3.88
99406	Behav chng smoking 3–10 min	14.91	11.86	0.24
99407	Behav chng smoking > 10 min	27.79	25.08	0.5
99415	Prolng clin staff svc 1st hour	18.98	18.98	0
99416	Prolng clin staff svc ea add	8.81	8.81	0
99421	Ol dig e/m svc 5–10 min	14.91	12.88	0.25
99422	Ol dig e/m svc 11–20 min	29.48	25.42	0.5
99423	Ol dig e/m svc 21+ min	47.10	40.33	0.8
99441	Phone e/m phys/qhp 5–10 min	56.25	34.90	0.7
99442	Phone e/m phys/qhp 11–20 min	90.82	66.08	1.3
99443	Phone e/m phys/qhp 21–30 min	127.76	96.92	1.92
99468	Neonate crit care initial	894.96	894.96	18.46
99469	Neonate crit care subsq	387.33	387.33	7.99

Table 12.1 (Continued)

E/M code	Short description	Non-facility price ($)	Facility price ($)	Work RVU
99471	*Ped critical care initial*	774.32	774.32	15.98
99472	*Ped critical care subsq*	392.75	392.75	7.99
99475	*Ped crit care age 205 initial*	558.12	558.12	11.25
99476	*Ped crit care age 205 subs*	336.50	336.50	6.75
99477	*Init day hosp neonate care*	339.21	339.21	7
99478	*Lc lbw inf < 1500gm subsq*	133.52	133.52	2.75
99479	*Lc lbw if 1500–2500g subsq*	121.66	121.66	2.5
99480	*Lc inf pbw 2501–5000g subsq*	117.25	117.25	2.4
99497	*Advncd care plan 30 min*	83.02	75.57	1.5
99498	*Advncd care plan addl 30 min*	71.84	71.50	1.4

Based on 2023 physician fee schedule https://www.cms.gov/medicare/physician-fee-schedule/search

INDEX

Note: *Italic* page numbers refer to figures.

Printed in the United States
by Baker & Taylor Publisher Services